Clinics in Developmental Medicine No. 175
PAEDIATRIC ORTHOTICS

© 2007 Mac Keith Press
30 Furnival Street, London EC4A 1JQ

Editor: Hilary M. Hart
Managing Editor: Michael Pountney
Project Manager: Edward Fenton

First published in this edition 2007

British Library Cataloguing-in-Publication data
A catalogue record for this book is available from the British Library

ISSN: 0069 4835
ISBN: 978 189 8683513

Typeset by Keystroke, 28 High Street, Tettenhall, Wolverhampton
Printed by The Lavenham Press Ltd, Water Street, Lavenham, Suffolk
Mac Keith Press is supported by Scope

Clinics in Developmental Medicine No. 175

Paediatric Orthotics

Edited by

CHRISTOPHER MORRIS, MSc, DPhil
Principal Orthotist, Nuffield Orthopaedic Centre;
MRC Training Fellow in Health Services Research, Department of
Public Health, University of Oxford &, Junior Research Fellow,
Wolfson College, Oxford, UK

Orthopaedic Editor

LUCIANO S. DIAS, MD
Professor of Orthopaedic Surgery, Northwestern University;
Medical Director, Motion Analysis Center, Children's Memorial
Hospital, Chicago, USA

2007
Mac Keith Press

Distributed by Blackwell Publishing

ACKNOWLEDGEMENT

We are extremely grateful to all our contributing authors and to Ed Fenton for his careful copy editing in the preparation of this book. We would also like to thank Hilary Hart, Martin Bax, David Scrutton, Michael Pountney and all at MacKeith Press for their encouragement and assistance in completing the project.

C.M. (Oxford) & L.D. (Chicago), 2007

CONTENTS

AUTHORS' APPOINTMENTS

Brigid Driscoll

Senior Physical Therapist and Orthotist, Children's Memorial Hospital, Chicago, USA

Trevor da Silva

Orthotist, The Hospital for Sick Children, Toronto, Canada

Michael El-Shammaa

Biomedical Engineer, Motion Analysis Center, Children's Memorial Hospital, Chicago, USA

Nicholas Gryfakis

Biomedical Engineer & Manager, Motion Analysis Center, Children's Memorial Hospital, Chicago, USA

Paul Horwood

Principal Orthotist, Nuffield Orthopaedic Centre, Oxford UK

Sheila Kellner

Certified Orthotist, Bloorview Kid's Rehab, Toronto, Canada

Robert Novak

Kinesiologist & Orthotist, Children's Memorial Hospital, Chicago, USA

Nicole M. Parent-Weiss

Orthotist & UH Satellite Team Leader, University of Michigan Orthotics and Prosthetics Center, Michigan, USA

Stephen Porter

Orthotist & Director, John Florence Ltd, Sussex, UK

Nicola Thompson

Physiotherapist & Clinical Specialist in Gait Analysis, Nuffield Orthopaedic Centre, Oxford, UK

FOREWORD

Many health professionals who care for children find themselves with a question about the need for orthotic management either in isolation or as part of the overall care of the child with a complex disability. It can be difficult as a general paediatrician, physiotherapist or orthopaedic surgeon to know where to access contemporary advice on orthotic management. What orthoses are available for this condition? How do they work? When should they be used? Will they be a stand-alone treatment or part of a medical and surgical intervention? Many of us feel that we know a little about orthotic practice and how it impinges on our work. Most of us, however, will confess to significant gaps in our knowledge. This book will fill a void, and will provide a handy reference for such moments.

Christopher Morris and Luciano Dias have assembled an excellent group of contributors including orthotists (practising and academic), biomedical engineers, physiotherapists and surgeons. An introductory chapter and a summary of biomechanical principles, by Dr Morris, are followed by practical information on assessment, materials, components and fabrication. There then follows an orderly presentation of upper-limb orthoses, lower-limb orthoses and their application to congenital deformities, acquired conditions and the challenging chronic physical disabilities of cerebral palsy, muscular dystrophies and myelo-meningocoele. Practical chapters on the orthotic management of scoliosis and protective and corrective headwear complete the book.

The references to each chapter are helpful but it is concerning to note the limited evidence base for many of the most common indications. This will surely point the discerning reader to many areas for further reflection and research. In the meantime this text is required reading for orthotists, biomedical engineers, physiotherapists, orthopaedic surgeons and many others involved in the care of children with musculoskeletal conditions including congenital abnormalities, physical disabilities and many acquired conditions.

H. Kerr Graham MD, FRCS (Ed), FRACS
Professor of Orthopaedic Surgery
The University of Melbourne
The Royal Children's Hospital

1
INTRODUCTION

Christopher Morris

Orthoses are externally applied medical devices used to modify the structural and functional characteristics of the neuromuscular and skeletal systems; orthoses work by applying forces to the body (International Organization for Standardization 1989a). Orthotists are health-care professionals trained in the clinical assessment, design and fitting of orthoses; they also have an educational background in bioengineering and the medical sciences. The role of the orthotist is to translate treatment goals into biomechanical objectives and then to design and fabricate an appropriate orthosis. At the fitting stage, the orthotist will ensure that the orthosis meets the biomechanical objectives; and once the orthosis has been supplied, the orthotist and the team will evaluate whether it succeeds in achieving the treatment goal. The orthotist also has a consultative role as part of the multidisciplinary team to advise or educate their colleagues about the use of orthoses.

The World Health Organization's International Classification of Functioning, Disability and Health (ICF) distinguishes between (1) body functions and structures, and (2) activities and participation as components of health (World Health Organization, 2001). In the terms used in the ICF, orthoses are designed to affect the body functions and structures, such as improving gait or preventing deformities, and to overcome activity limitations and participation restrictions by enabling people to have more involvement in life situations. As will be seen in this book an orthosis is frequently designed to achieve all these aims. This book aims to describe the contribution that orthoses can make to the physical management of children. In *Chapter 2* we outline the fundamental biomechanical principles that underpin orthotic design. Then, in *Chapter 3*, we consider the process of clinical assessment relevant for orthotic management, with a special emphasis on gait analysis; this is because lower-limb orthoses are frequently used with the goal of improving gait patterns. *Chapter 4* describes some of the materials, components and fabrication techniques that are used to construct orthoses in the context of the orthotic supply process. The introductory chapters end with *Chapters 5* and *6*, which respectively catalogue the various types of upper- and lower-limb orthoses. Then, in the second section of the book, several chapters consider the orthotic management of some of the more common conditions. In *Chapter 7* we record orthotic intervention for some of the congenital anomalies with which children are born, and in *Chapter 8* we consider the treatment of a selection of different conditions in which symptoms arise during childhood. Three common neuromuscular conditions requiring orthotic intervention are cerebral palsy, which is dealt with in *Chapter 9*; the muscular dystrophies, atrophies and peripheral neuropathies, which are covered in *Chapter 10*; and myelomeningocoele, dealt with in *Chapter 11*. The management of scoliosis not due to those conditions is described in *Chapter 12*; finally, in *Chapter 13*, we consider orthoses used to protect the head and more recently potentially to remodel head shape in infants. The remainder of this introduction outlines the terminology used to name orthoses and considers briefly how orthotics has evolved over the recent decades with the availability of new materials.

Terminology

The term *orthosis* (plural: orthoses) may have superseded other terms such *brace* or *splint* amongst some health professionals, as similarly the term *orthotist* has replaced 'appliance fitter'. We have deliberately tried to avoid using the terms *brace*, *splint* and *calliper* in this book. However, the terms used to describe various orthoses continue to be inconsistent. The use of acronyms proliferates in the field and it can often be difficult to know what these abbreviations really mean. Similarly, the term *dynamic* is often used inconsistently to describe a variety of orthoses, and this expression should generally be avoided. Three systems for naming orthoses are most commonly used: anatomical, functional and nominal.

ANATOMICAL

The correct terminology for describing an orthosis is generally accepted to be an indication of the joints that a device encompasses (International Organization for Standardization 1989b). Hence an ankle–foot orthosis (AFO), for example, extends from below the knee to include the ankle and foot, and a knee–ankle–foot orthosis (KAFO) would extend more proximally to the thigh and include the knee joint. Orthoses may be designed to affect the hip joint only (HpO), or be part of more complex devices such as hip–knee–ankle–foot orthoses (HKAFOs), or be used in conjunction with thoracolumbar–sacral–spinal orthoses (TLSOs). Note that the acronym HpO is used for hip orthoses to distinguish these from hand orthoses (HdOs).

FUNCTIONAL

Aside from anatomical coverage it is also useful to know what effect the orthosis is designed to achieve. For this reason, descriptive terms such as 'hip-abduction spinal sitting orthosis' (HASSO) and 'cranial remoulding orthosis' have also been adopted.

NOMINAL

Naming orthoses after people or places is commonplace but confusing and therefore this practice should in general be avoided. However, although it is generally preferable to use anatomical nomenclature to communicate unambiguously, especially in academic literature, a few eponymous titles or trade names are included in this text where it is otherwise unavoidable to refer to specific orthoses.

Historical aspects

The introduction of modular components and plastics has largely made redundant many of the traditional skills of orthotists and technicians who once hand-forged metals using blacksmith-style forges. Contemporary lightweight plastic orthoses have proved a major advance from conventional orthoses made from metal substructures and finished with what might now be considered elaborate leatherwork. However, orthotics has changed relatively slowly in comparison with other realms of orthopaedic and rehabilitation technologies which have successfully exploited even lighter composite materials and computer-aided design and manufacturing processes. Despite their apparent simplicity, orthoses continue to play an important role in the physical management of childhood disability. As can be seen in the condition-specific chapters, orthoses enable children to sit, stand and walk, and therefore to experience and participate in life more fully than otherwise might be possible.

This book is intended to be useful as a reference both for orthotists and other health professionals who want to know more about the utility of orthoses in improving the care of children with neuromuscular and musculoskeletal diagnoses. Alongside the key technical aspects of orthotic management, it is important to incorporate the orthotist as a member any paediatric neuromuscular multidisciplinary team, and to ensure that the service is delivered in a family-centred way. Finally, we emphasize the need to monitor clinical outcomes; the aim of intervention should be to improve the child's health and well-being and not simply to solve biomechanical problems.

References

International Organization for Standardization (1989a) *ISO 8549-1 Prosthetics and Orthotics – Vocabulary, Part 1: General Terms for External Limb Prostheses and External Orthoses*. Geneva: ISO.
International Organization for Standardization (1989b) *ISO 8549-3 Prosthetics and Orthotics – Vocabulary, Part 3: Terms Relating to External Orthoses*. Geneva: ISO.
World Health Organization (2001) *International Classification of Functioning, Disability and Health*. Geneva: WHO.

2
BIOMECHANICAL PRINCIPLES

Christopher Morris

By definition, orthoses work by applying forces to the body. Therefore in order to understand the principles of orthotic management it is necessary to have at least a rudimentary appreciation of the mechanics of structures and the way they interact with the body, i.e. *biomechanics*. The first step in learning about the application of mechanics to the body is to consider the body as a system of rigid segments, hinged at joints and linked by muscles and ligaments. The angle between these segments is altered or controlled through the action of external forces (gravitational, environmental or orthotic) or internal forces (muscular, ligamentous or inertial).

Forces and vectors

Forces are *vector* quantities, that is they have both magnitude and direction. A single force acting on an object causes motion in the direction of the applied force. However, two forces acting on an object can cause compression, tension, shear or turning, and three forces can cause bending, depending on the direction in which the forces are acting (Fig. 2.1). When two forces are acting in different planes at right angles to each other, then the magnitude and line of action of their combined effect can be calculated using geometry, and this is called the *resultant force*. Similarly, the magnitude of a single force acting in any direction can be converted (*resolved*) into its vertical and horizontal components (Fig. 2.2).

Reaction forces

All objects are affected by gravity. An object pushes down on the ground with a force (its weight) equal to its mass multiplied by gravity. Isaac Newton stated that for every action there is an equal and opposite reaction. Therefore a surface supporting an object in equilibrium, for example the ground supporting the body, pushes back with a reaction force equal to the weight (its mass multiplied by gravity) of the object (Fig. 2.3). Although we are not usually aware of it, the ground pushes back under our feet by being compressed minutely until it generates a force equal to our weight. One can see this more clearly when standing on a trampoline which distorts until it can generate a reaction force equal to the body's weight. Whilst this concept is straightforward when a body is static, during motion the reaction force on a body acts in all three planes. Using geometry, however, it can still be calculated as the resultant *ground reaction force* if the vertical and horizontal components are known (Fig. 2.4). Nearly all forces applied by orthoses are *reaction forces*. Orthoses usually oppose forces applied to them by the body as a result of gravity, hypertonia, muscle imbalance or inertial forces, and in doing so they oppose changes in body posture.

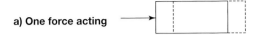

a) One force acting

Fig. 2.1 Different ways in which forces can act on an object: (a) one force, (b) two forces, and (c) three forces.

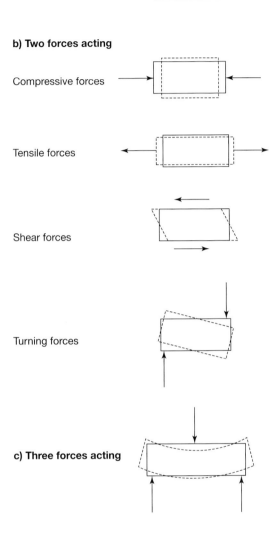

b) Two forces acting

Compressive forces

Tensile forces

Shear forces

Turning forces

c) Three forces acting

Occasionally orthoses do apply *active forces* by incorporating springs, elastics or compressed gas pistons into the device, and these release the stored energy when those components are deformed.

Moments and levers

Forces acting around a fulcrum create a turning effect called the *moment*. Moments in any direction can be calculated from the magnitude of the force multiplied by the perpendicular distance at which the force is acting from the fulcrum point. This is why we push doors on

5

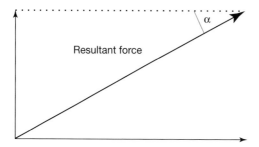

Resultant force

α

Fig. 2.2 The magnitude and direction of the resultant force of two forces acting at a right angle to each other can be calculated using geometry. Similarly, the magnitude of a single force acting in any direction can be resolved into its vertical and horizontal components.

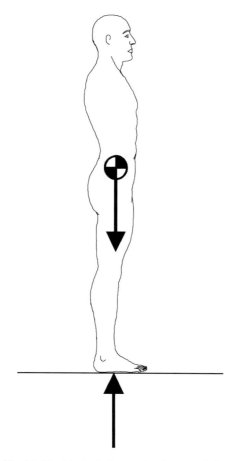

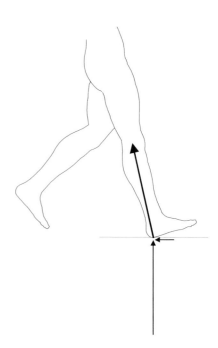

Fig. 2.3 The total body force acting downwards from its centre of mass is resisted by an equal and opposite reaction force from the support surface, following Newton's Third Law.

Fig. 2.4 At initial contact, the horizontal and vertical reaction forces create a resultant ground reaction force (GRF). The line of action of the GRF can affect moments around proximal joints, but it usually remains close to the hip and knee joints during normal gait.

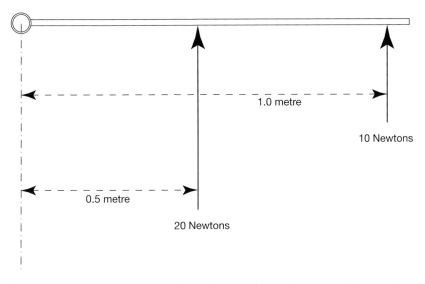

1.0 metre

10 Newtons

0.5 metre

20 Newtons

Fig. 2.5 A smaller force acting at a greater distance from the fulcrum, in this case a hinge on a door, will produce an equal moment to a greater force applied at a shorter distance (10 Newton metres in both cases). With equal forces, therefore, the longer the lever arm, the greater the moment generated.

the side furthest from the hinges, because the force required to open them is reduced (Fig. 2.5). To prevent turning, the moments acting in one direction must be balanced by the moments acting in the other direction. This is the principle of the children's see-saw (or teeter-totter), where moments acting in one direction due to a force acting at a distance on one side of the fulcrum can be balanced by an equal moment acting in the opposite direction. The further a force acts from the fulcrum (measured at right angles to the direction of the force), the less force is required to generate a moment; conversely, the shorter the distance, the greater the force required to generate an equal moment (Fig. 2.6).

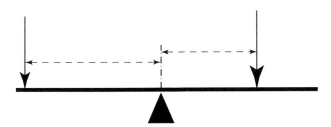

Fig. 2.6 Moments acting in one direction on one side of the fulcrum are balanced by the moments acting in the other direction on the opposite side of the fulcrum (Moment = $10 \times 1.5 = 15 \times 1 = 15$ Newton metres). Note that the shorter the distance from the fulcrum at which the force acts (lever arm), the greater the magnitude of force required to generate the same moment.

7

The levers described so far were long and straight and acted in a single plane, similar to the femur and tibia either side of the knee joint. However, when considering the hip joint (for instance), the pelvis is irregular in shape and the joint moves in all three planes, and to complicate matters further, one hip joint cannot usually be considered separately from the spine and the opposite hip. Similarly, the spine consists of relatively small segments, corresponding to each vertebra lying deep under subcutaneous tissue. Therefore controlling body segments such as the pelvis and spine poses much more complex challenges for the orthotist than distal joints.

Stress and strain

The diagrams in Figure 2.1 show how forces can deform objects in various ways as a result of compression, tension, shear or turning, and bending, which involves both compression and tension. The ratio of change in dimension of an object with respect to the original dimensions describes the concept known as *strain*, and has no unit of measurement. *Stress*, on the other hand, describes the amount of force applied to an object as a function of the area of its application, and can be measured as the force per unit area in 'Newtons per square metre' or Pascals.

Stiffness and strength

For many materials, the incremental application of a force producing stress creates a proportional increase in strain (Fig. 2.7). Different gradients of relationship between stress and strain indicate the stiffness of a material. Materials with high stiffness require large amounts of stress to produce even small amounts of strain, whereas less stiff materials are susceptible to large amounts of strain with relatively small amounts of stress. Whilst the relationship between stress and strain remains linear, the deformation is known as *elastic* as the object will return to its previous size and shape when the stress is removed. For materials that demonstrate *elastic* deformation the relationship stress and strain is a measure of its stiffness and is known as Young's modulus (E). The term *viscoelastic* is often used to describe materials such as silicon rubbers that can be deformed in any direction and still return to their original dimensions.

Strength

The concept of strength represents the amount of stress required to cause a material or object to fail during a single loading. In contrast to elastic deformation, permanent or *plastic* deformation occurs when the relationship between stress and strain becomes non-linear (Fig. 2.7). This change in the material's behaviour occurs at the *yield point*, and following this point the material will no longer return to its unloaded size and shape when the stress is removed. Materials that undergo plastic deformation prior to fracture are known as *ductile*, whilst materials that fail suddenly during elastic deformation are known as *brittle*. The relevance of these issues to orthotic design is that by using ductile materials we should have some warning prior to catastrophic failure. In fact, as the energy required to cause failure is represented by the area under the curves in Figure 2.7, ductile materials also require many times the amount of energy to fracture. Further consideration of these concepts in relation

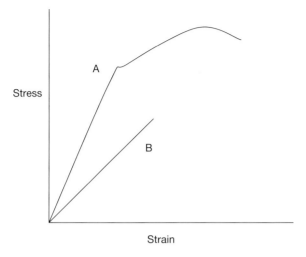

Fig. 2.7 Stress–strain curve indicating the stiffness and strength of materials. After initial elastic deformation, *curve A* represents a ductile material where after a yield point there is a period of plastic deformation prior to failure; *curve B* shows a brittle material that fails without warning.

to the specific materials commonly used in orthotics is provided in the next chapter, as they are often also affected by methods of fabrication and the number of times an object can be expected to be loaded.

Bending

When three forces act on an object as in Figure 2.8, the moments generated may cause bending. The resistance of the object to bending is dependent on its material and cross-sectional area and the distribution of the material about the bending axis. The bending

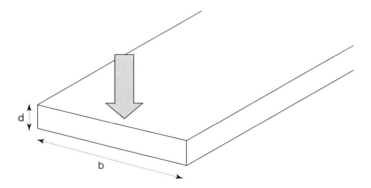

Fig. 2.8 An object's resistance to bending is dependent on its cross-sectional area and the distribution of the material about the bending axis. The bending resistance of a beam is known as the *second moment of area* (I).

9

resistance of an object such as a beam is known as the *second moment of area* (I) and increases in proportion to its thickness cubed (d^3), and directly with increases in its width (b) (Fig. 2.8). The importance of material distribution to resist bending can be demonstrated by first flexing a plastic ruler across its flat plane, and then again after rotating it 90° along its axis. The ruler will allow large deflection about the flat plane whereas it is not possible to notice any deflection having rotated it, even though the cross-sectional area is the same. The length of an object such as a lever or beam will also influence its resistance to bending. As we have seen, the greater the distance a force is applied from the supporting points, the greater the moments that will be generated; but there will also be greater bending with increasing length. When designing structures to resist bending, the distance between the supporting points will influence the size and shape of the cross-sectional area and the choice of material. It is also more efficient to have the material distributed as far from the bending axis as possible, such as in the I-shaped metal girders used in buildings.

Pressure
Forces acting on an object must have an area over which they are applied. The pressure on the surface of the object is proportional to the size of the area over which the force acts. The larger the contact area then the lower the pressure created at the contact surface. Needles and nails have very small contact areas so that even with the application of low forces the pressure is sufficient to penetrate objects. A drawing-pin has both a sharp end, with a tiny contact point, and a larger contact area for us to push. Soft cushions are used on hard chairs as these deform to increase the contact surface area and hence appreciably decrease the pressure and improve the comfort of sitting. Sustained excessive pressure on the body leads to localised ischemia and tissue breakdown in the form of pressure sores. Hence padding is often added inside orthoses over bony areas which are more prone to high pressure.

Friction
Friction describes the amount of resistance that occurs when one object attempts to slide over another. The amount of friction between two objects depends largely upon the contact surfaces of the adjacent objects. For instance, ice is smoother than tarmac and therefore one needs to be more cautious when walking on it. It is usually safer to take shorter steps on an icy surface because it increases friction by reducing the horizontal components of the ground reaction force. Outdoors, for safety and to improve propulsion, we often need to increase friction between the orthosis and the ground, and so we use rubber materials on the soles of shoes or the tips of walking aids. However in orthotic hinges we want low friction articulations to increase mechanical efficiency. At the orthosis–body interface, friction creates the risk of rubbing and tissue damage in the forms of blisters.

Stability
Stability describes the relationship between the position of the centre of mass (often called the centre of gravity) and its base of support. The distribution of material that constitutes an object influences the position of the centre of mass of that object. The weight of the object is its mass multiplied by gravity, and it acts vertically downward from the centre of

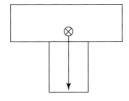

Fig. 2.9 Stability is defined by the relationship between the line of force from the centre of mass of an object and its base of support. (a) When the line from the centre of mass falls within the base of support then stability is achieved. (b) When the line from the centre of mass falls outside the base of support, then the object is unstable. (c) Maximum stability is achieved with a wide base of support and low centre of gravity.

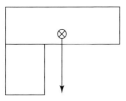

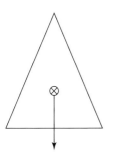

mass. When the line from the centre of mass falls within the base of support then stability is achieved. However, when the line from the centre of mass falls outside the base of support, then the object is unstable (Fig. 2.9). Stability can be increased by having a wide base of support, as in the Eiffel Tower for example, and by keeping the centre of mass as low as possible. Stability has a strong influence on the amount of energy necessary to initiate movement. The more stable an object is, the greater the energy required to generate movement. Maximum stability may be desirable in some circumstances, such as when using orthotic frames designed to enable standing; but when any movement is desirable, stability may need to be compromised to enable energy-efficient locomotion.

Summary

This chapter has described the basic biomechanical principles that are fundamental to designing orthoses. Most orthoses work using a combination of three point force systems (Fig. 2.1c) and by manipulating the ground reaction force to react to forces generated by the body and its interaction with the environment. In general, effective orthoses utilize the maximum length of leverage (to reduce the magnitude of the force required) and then apply the force over the largest possible surface area to reduce the pressure between the orthosis and the body.

Further reading

Gordon JE (1991) *Structures: Or Why Things Don't Fall Down*. Harmondsworth, UK: Penguin.

3
ASSESSMENT

Christopher Morris, Nicholas Gryfakis, Michael El-Shammaa and Luciano Dias

A careful assessment of the child's needs is essential if orthotic management is to be successful and to avoid unnecessarily adding problems to the child's or family's lives. Prescription of orthoses is only one mode of physical management, and it should not be considered separately from other surgical or therapeutic interventions. Therefore physical management planning may, at times, require input from the broad multidisciplinary team including paediatrician, physical and occupational therapist, physiatrist, orthopaedic surgeon, orthotist, psychologist, social worker and others as appropriate. The assessment will require taking a medical history, identifying the child's physical and functional problems by examining the range of movement in their joints, their selective muscle control and strength. Further investigations such as radiological studies and instrumented gait analysis may be necessary to understand problems not discernible or detected by observation alone. The assessment establishes the treatment goals and, if an orthosis is to be provided, the biomechanical objective for that orthosis; only then can an appropriate orthosis be designed. Whatever the treatment goals a family-centred approach will encourage compliance with the prescribed treatment regimen (King et al. 1996). The team must therefore be well coordinated, work in partnership with the family, and provide adequate information about the condition, the role of interventions and their expected outcomes (Rosenbaum et al. 1992). Before measuring and making any orthosis, therefore, it is necessary to understand the child's and family's perception of the problems and to ensure their aspirations for the outcome of treatment are realistic.

Supply process
There is a logical sequence to the orthotic supply process, and Figure 3.1 (modified from Condie and Stewart 1997) shows the key elements and who should be involved at each stage. Assessment by the team, ideally involving the orthotist, results in a prescription for an orthosis. The referral must include all the information about the child's diagnosis, treatment goals targeted, biomechanical problem, and the name of the recommended orthosis if known. Once a specific design of orthosis is agreed with the team, the orthotist can set about taking the measurements and if required taking a cast model of the relevant body segments and writing the specification. Then the orthotist and orthotic technicians can manufacture the orthosis ready for delivery; occasionally, for some complex orthoses, a trial fitting is undertaken before the orthosis is finished.

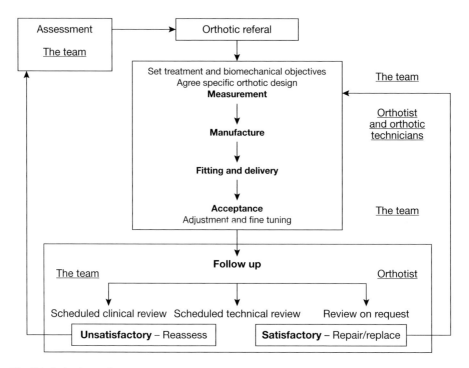

Fig. 3.1 Orthotic supply process.

The family must be provided with instructions on how and when to use the orthosis at the time of final fitting and supply. All the members of the team then need to encourage the child and family towards acceptance of the orthosis; allowing the child to choose the colour or pattern of their orthosis at the measuring stage is helpful to achieve this aim. Subsequently there must be an evaluation of whether the orthosis has solved the biomechanical problem and most importantly enabled the treatment goals to be achieved. Further follow-up with the orthotist is often necessary for fine-tuning of the orthosis or modification if it is uncomfortable. These appointments shortly after supply should not be delayed if at all possible as this creates long periods when the orthosis is not being used. Later, ensuring ready access and regular review appointments with the orthotist will ensure the safety of the orthosis and allow for any repair or replacement of the orthosis. Ideally repairs should be undertaken on the day so that the child is not left without any orthosis; this is much easier to achieve if appropriate workshop facilities are available. In general, regular clinical review with the team will ensure the prescribed orthosis remains appropriate and also allow consideration of whether any other intervention might be required.

Factors affecting prescription
The appropriate plan for treating each child will be influenced by the type and severity of their impairments, their individual activity limitations and their goals. The effectiveness

of any treatment will also be influenced by the availability of adjuvant physical therapy and the family's motivation.

RANGE OF MOVEMENT

Orthoses commonly try to impose a posture in some part of the body; it is therefore essential that that posture is realistic (i.e. possible to achieve) and tolerable to the child. Orthoses are often reputed to be uncomfortable and to cause rubbing or soreness; however, these problems can be avoided through careful assessment of joint flexibility and the range of motion present. One important rule is that you can only achieve with an orthosis what you can achieve with your hands; trying to impose unrealistic correction of deformities is one reason why discomfort and skin breakdown occur.

A paediatric orthopaedic surgeon and physical therapist will be helpful for a thorough physical examination, but a few key tests of range of movement are commonly used to assess for orthotic intervention. The range of dorsiflexion available at the ankle affects lower-limb function and the efficacy of any ankle–foot or foot orthosis. As the gastrocnemius muscle crosses both the knee and ankle joints, range of motion at the ankle can vary with the degree of knee flexion; dorsiflexion should therefore be assessed with the knee flexed and also with the knee fully extended.

MUSCLE CONTROL AND STRENGTH

An assessment of which muscle groups are functioning and capable of generating useful power, and which muscles the child has selective control over, is crucial in the planning of orthotic intervention. Orthoses are used both to compensate for weak muscles and also to oppose any inappropriate muscle activity. Simple grading systems such as the MRC scale for grading muscle strength, which ranges from 0 (indicating no active movement) to 5 (for full strength), are used to record muscle strength. However, more reliable measurement of muscle strength can be undertaken using dynamometry.

JOINT CONGRUENCY AND INTEGRITY

The integrity of the child's skeleton can be assessed through radiological studies to highlight any bony or joint abnormalities. X-rays are particularly useful in the assessment of scoliosis and can be used as blueprints to design the orthosis. X-rays may also be used to check whether an orthosis is achieving its intended biomechanical effect, for instance when using a hip-abduction orthosis to position the femoral head in the acetabulum.

SENSATION

Some conditions, such as myelomeningocoele and hereditary motor sensory neuropathy, reduce the child's ability to feel sensations on the skin. It is important to take this into account as the child may then not be aware of excessive pressure caused by an orthosis and there is a risk that pressure sores can occur without the usual forewarning signals.

Children requiring orthotic management often have complex diagnoses and are receiving help for other impairments. These may be unrelated to the reasons for orthotic treatment but it is nonetheless important to take them into account. For instance, following gastrostomy, the need to provide access for feeding tubes is an important consideration for a spinal orthosis. There may be more pressing medical problems which take precedence over the need for an orthosis. It can also be necessary to take account of factors such as hearing or vision loss, intellectual ability, seizures, and the child's mode of communication.

Gait analysis

Human gait is a complex reciprocal motion. When analyzing gait, it is important to be able to reference key events. Thus gait is described according to the gait cycle (GC); this is defined from initial foot contact with the ground to the next consecutive initial contact on the same side and is equivalent to one stride. The gait cycle can then be divided into two main phases: stance and swing. Stance is considered the first phase of the gait cycle and swing is considered the second and last phase of the gait cycle. In order to enable intra- and inter-patient comparisons, the gait cycle can also be described in terms of percentage. In normal gait, stance phase occurs from 0% to 60% of the gait cycle and swing phase occurs from 60% to 100%.

Stance phase can be further divided into five periods: initial contact, loading response, mid stance, terminal stance, and pre-swing. Initial contact (0% GC) is the instant at which the foot makes contact with the floor. One may also see initial contact described as foot contact or heel strike; however these terms are not general enough to be applied to all gait patterns seen in various pathologies. At this point of the gait cycle, the contralateral foot is still in contact with the ground. Loading response (0%–10% GC) occurs from initial contact until the contralateral foot has left the ground, otherwise known as opposite foot off. This period can also be described as double support phase or double limb stance. Mid-stance (10%–30% GC) occurs from the end of loading response until the point when the body has progressed over and in front of the stance foot. Terminal stance (30%–50% GC) begins at the end of mid-stance and continues until initial contact of the opposite foot. Mid-stance and terminal stance combined (10%–50% GC) constitute the period of single limb support. Pre-swing (50%–60% GC) begins at the end of terminal stance and continues until the foot has left the ground (foot-off). The time when the ipsilateral foot has left the ground is often referred to as toe-off, but for the same reasons as listed above, its generality is not sufficient. This period of pre-swing can also be described as terminal double limb stance, as the contralateral foot is in contact in the floor. The foot-off event constitutes the end of the stance phase of gait. An illustration of the stance phase of gait is shown in Figure 3.2.

Swing phase can be divided into three periods: initial, mid- and terminal swing. Initial swing (60%–73% GC) begins at the end of pre-swing and continues until the swinging foot is opposite the contralateral foot on the floor. Mid-swing (73%–87% GC) begins at the end of initial swing and concludes when the swinging tibia becomes vertical relative to the ground. Finally, terminal swing (87%–100% GC) occurs from the end of mid-swing until initial contact is made once again. An illustration of the swing phase of gait is shown in

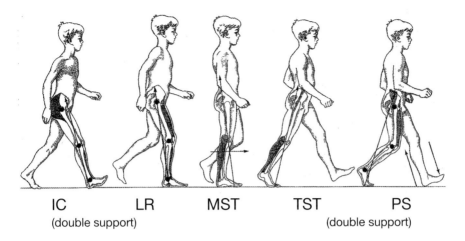

IC   LR   MST   TST   PS
(double support)   (double support)

Fig. 3.2 The stance phase of gait and its five subdivisions: initial contact (IC), loading response (LR), mid-stance (MST), terminal stance (TST) and pre-swing (PS). (From Gage 2004, by permission.)

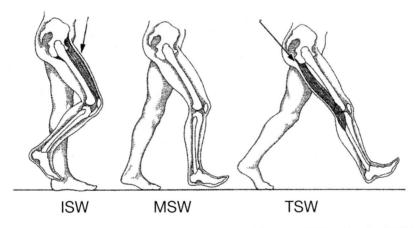

ISW   MSW   TSW

Fig. 3.3 The swing phase of gait and its three subdivisions: initial swing (ISW), mid-swing (MSW) and terminal swing (TSW). (From Gage 2004, by permission.)

Figure 3.3. The end of terminal swing defines the end of one gait cycle. Due to the reciprocal nature of gait, as soon as one gait cycle ends for the ipsilateral limb, the next cycle begins until the cessation of walking. Furthermore, the ipsilateral and contralateral gait cycles occur simultaneously but out of phase with each other (Sutherland 1988, Perry 1992).

GAIT PARAMETERS
Several measurements can be made based on the phases and periods of the gait cycle. Common temporal measurements include: stride length, step length, walking velocity and

17

cadence. Stride length is defined as the distance travelled by one foot in one gait cycle. Step length is defined as the distance between each foot during consecutive double support phases; hence a stride is made up of two consecutive steps. Cadence is the frequency of steps taken during gait and is typically reported as the number of steps per minute. Walking velocity is the average distance travelled in a period of time and is calculated by dividing the stride length by the time duration of the stride. Walking velocity can be reported as an absolute measure (metres per second) or as a normalized percentage of an age-matched comparison.

OBSERVATIONAL GAIT ANALYSIS

Observational gait analysis involves watching the individual walking; the observer documents what s/he sees, based on experience and expertise. Observational gait analysis allows the clinician to assess the overall smoothness of the gait pattern and any gross abnormalities that are present. Each child's movement pattern can be visually compared to the observer's perception of what is normal and rated as normal, slightly abnormal or significantly abnormal. The reliability and accuracy of information gained from this method has a strong relationship with level of expertise of the observer. Unfortunately clinic layouts often restrict the planes of observation available to the clinician as children are often asked to walk in hallways or corridors.

A more reliable method than simply watching the child in clinic involves video gait analysis. Two cameras are often used so that motion can be simultaneously viewed in both the sagittal and frontal planes; in principle the transverse plane can be viewed using an overhead camera but this is uncommon. Filming gait allows the observer to repeatedly view the gait of the child in real time or slow motion and to focus on the global ambulation pattern or a specific part of the body. The assessment of foot pathology during gait is often assessed using biplanar close-up video and foot-pressure analysis. The slower the video is played back, the greater consistency of the assessment for single and multiple observers (Krebs et al. 1985, Brunnekreef et al. 2005). Video can be recorded whilst the child is wearing and not wearing an orthosis and then compared subjectively.

The observational method has weaknesses however, even using video, as cross-planar motions impair the observer's ability to accurately quantify joint angles. For example, knee flexion can be misinterpreted as knee valgus if there is femoral anteversion, an increased range of pelvic or hip rotation or if the camera is not properly aligned to the plane of motion (Fig. 3.4). Furthermore, evaluation of proximal segments using video can be difficult if there is excessive soft tissue around the trunk, pelvis and hips obscures motion (Gage 2004). Observational gait analysis, even with video, is widely used as it is inexpensive and can provide quick feedback.

INSTRUMENTED THREE-DIMENSIONAL GAIT ANALYSIS

Instrumented three-dimensional (3D) gait analysis is restricted to a controlled laboratory setting. The most common 3D gait analysis systems use passive markers which reflect light coming from special cameras (Fig. 3.5), although other systems use electromagnetic sensors or active light-emitting markers. The locations of the markers in space are captured via a

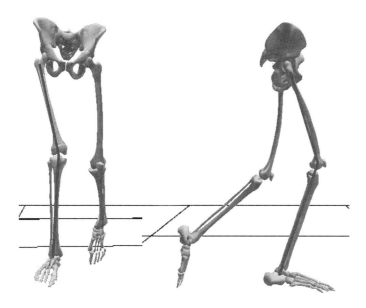

Fig. 3.4 Knee flexion and internal rotation can be misinterpreted as knee valgus when only 2D observational analysis is used.

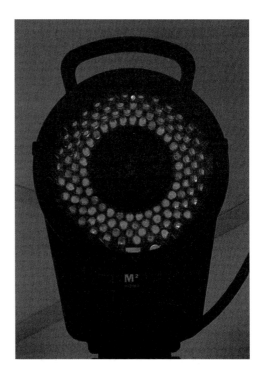

Fig. 3.5 Specialized 3D motion analysis camera with light-emitting strobes around the camera lens.

multiple camera system and digital processors. Typical motion-capture systems include six to twelve cameras placed strategically around the room; the system calculates the 3D coordinates of each marker in the laboratory space providing the marker is visible to at least two cameras. Hence the greater the number of cameras the less the risk of markers being lost to the system.

The markers are placed on the child's body on specific anatomical landmarks according to a standard procedure based on a biomechanical model. The model utilizes the 3D position coordinates of each marker together with anthropometric measurements to calculate the major joint centres and angles instantaneously during the gait cycle. Joint angles are calculated in an ordered series, usually from proximal to distal segments in the sagittal, coronal and transverse planes. The instrumented method therefore provides more accurate calculations of joint angles compared to observational and video gait analysis. Graphical plots are generated which display the joint angles relative to the gait cycle allowing objective intra-child consistency comparisons as well as comparisons to a normal database. These plots of the joint angles during gait are called kinematic data and are interpreted together with the temporal parameters such as walking velocity, cadence, step length, and stride length.

Force plates are frequently used simultaneously with 3D systems, enabling the ground reaction forces to be captured during stance phase. Information about the ground reaction force is used in conjunction with the kinematic data to calculate joint kinetics, which are the moments acting around joints during gait. Joint moments provide insight to the stresses placed on the joints. For instance, these data can be used to assess whether orthotic intervention reduces the frontal-plane knee moment compared to walking barefoot. Additionally, kinetic data allow one to calculate the power generated or absorbed during the gait cycle. For example, knee-power generation plots can provide the clinician with an understanding of the degree of concentric or eccentric muscle contraction occurring at different points of the gait cycle.

Instrumented 3D gait analysis is widely used as a tool to assess outcomes after interventions as well as an assessment tool to help guide the treatment of children with gait abnormalities. The data collection, interpretation and making of recommendations based on kinematic and kinetic data require a bioengineer, kinesiologist or physical therapist, orthotist and orthopaedic surgeon who are all experienced in 3D gait analysis. As a result of the requirement for skilled staff, the cost of buying and maintaining special equipment, and the length of time taken to collect data, 3D gait analysis is more expensive than observational or videotape gait analysis. Consequently, the appropriateness of undertaking 3D gait analysis depends upon the nature of the clinical question.

ELECTROMYOGRAPHY

Electromyography (EMG) uses electrodes to measure the electrical activity of muscles to determine the relative magnitude and timing of muscle contractions. There are two methods for obtaining EMG data, either using a surface-mounted electrode (Fig. 3.6) or with a fine-wire (needle) electrode (Fig. 3.7). Surface electrodes are placed on the skin over large muscles to measure the overall activity; a fine-wire electrode is pushed through the skin,

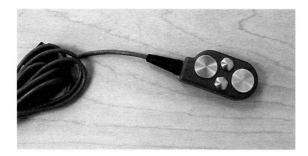

Fig. 3.6 Surface-mounted electrode.

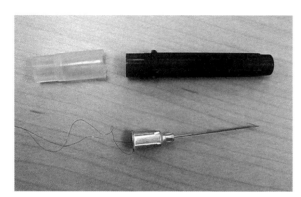

Fig. 3.7 Fine-wire (or needle) electrode.

and placed directly on or into the muscle to measure activity of specific muscles or motor units. Wireless EMG hardware can be used to improve portability of the system. The primary advantage of a surface mounted EMG is the ease of data collection; the electrode is secured to the skin with adhesive strips or collars to apply continuous pressure. Surface EMGs also have the advantage of not being painful and invasive, which makes it easier for children.

The main disadvantage with surface EMG is the relatively poor data quality compared with fine-wire methods. However, data quality can be adequate for many purposes although it should be interpreted with some caution. Surface EMG is also limited to only measuring activity of muscles that are near the surface and large enough to be covered by the electrode. Other factors that may affect data quality include appropriate positioning, skin movement and electrical interference; sweat, dirt particles, skin abnormalities and hair may also cause signal noise. Therefore it is often worth drying, cleaning and shaving the limb to improve data quality. The main advantage of the fine wire method is that it is capable of monitoring activity of deeper muscles such as posterior tibialis that cannot be assessed from the skin surface. The positioning of the fine-wire electrode can be tested by stimulating the muscle and is less susceptible to signal noise and interference.

Some of the muscles typically monitored with surface or fine-wire EMG during gait analysis include but are not limited to gastrocnemius, anterior tibialis, tibialis posterior, peroneus longus, vastus lateralis, vastus medialis, medial hamstrings, lateral hamstrings, rectus femoris, adductor longus, gluteus medius and gluteus maximus. The EMG hardware can record multiple electrode channels simultaneously which can then be synchronized with kinematic and kinetic data.

Once the EMGs are in position, the child can begin walking and the EMG activity recorded (Fig. 3.8) and normalized (Fig. 3.9) to the gait cycle, from heel contact to heel contact. The EMG signal is examined to assess data quality. There are several different methods for processing EMG data with filters and linear envelopes; however, raw data are often presented. Typically EMG data are displayed with the normal muscle-timing patterns on the bottom of the graph for comparison (shown as solid bar at the bottom of Fig. 3.9). EMG is useful to determine changes in muscle activity with and without different orthoses. For example, Park et al. (1997) showed that in patients with sacral-level myelomeningocoele there was increased stance-phase quadriceps activity when walking barefoot, which was significantly reduced with the use of solid ankle–foot orthoses (AFOs). Lam et al. (2005) showed that when children with cerebral palsy were wearing AFOs the median EMG frequency was decreased, suggesting increased walking endurance.

FOOT PRESSURE
Foot-pressure data are especially useful when assessing the effect of orthotic intervention. Foot-pressure analysis is used to show areas of increased or decreased pressure under the

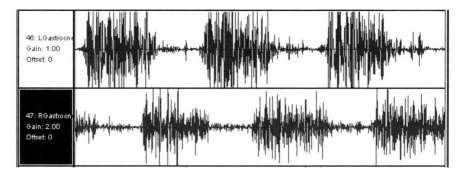

Fig. 3.8 Raw EMG data from three gait cycles of the left and right gastrocnemius.

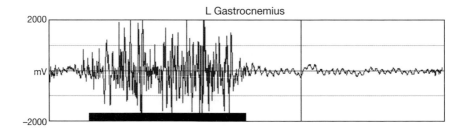

Fig. 3.9 Normalized EMG data from the left gastrocnemius, from foot contact to foot contact.

22

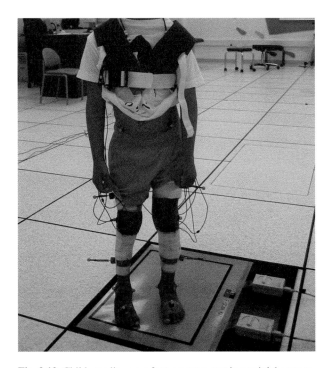

Fig. 3.10 Child standing on a foot-pressure mat in a gait laboratory.

foot; information which can guide modification of an orthosis. As pressure is a function of force divided by area, and the force due to body weight cannot be readily changed, pressure can best be decreased by increasing the surface area over which the force is applied. Foot-pressure analysis helps one to visualize this phenomenon and then to determine the best course of action. Foot-pressure data can be collected while the child is standing, walking or running barefoot using a pressure mat laid on the floor (as seen in Fig. 3.10); alternatively measurements can be taken within the shoe, using a thin insert placed between the foot and the orthosis or the insole of the shoe (Fig. 3.11). Foot-pressure data can be used to check the alignment and efficacy of an orthosis; for instance Figure 3.12 shows pressure data collected between a hinged AFO and the shoe as well as the pressure distribution between the foot and the orthosis, from a patient with a partial foot amputation. These data show that the alignment of the orthosis in the shoe is incorrect as all areas of peak pressure are on the lateral edge of the shoe. Incidentally, it was also noticed that the areas of peak pressure on the foot are at the same location as a callus, and where the patient was feeling pain.

It can be difficult to determine the exact location on the foot of increased pressure with a typical foot-pressure display (Fig. 3.13). A technique has been developed at the Motion Analysis Center at Children's Memorial Hospital (Chicago, IL, USA) that allows for a more beneficial display of foot-pressure data relative to the exact shape and size of the individual

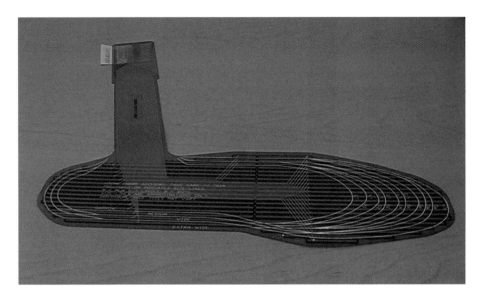

Fig. 3.11 An example of an in-shoe foot-pressure measuring system.

(a) (b)

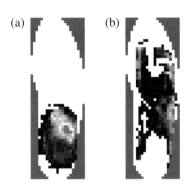

Fig. 3.12 Foot-pressure data collected for a patient with a partial foot amputation showing the difference in pressure distribution (a) between the foot and the orthosis and (b) between the orthosis and the shoe.

foot (Fig. 3.14). This allows the clinician to view foot pressure relative to anatomical landmarks on the individual foot. For example, it would be easy to see that an area of increased pressure is at the same spot on the foot as a callus. Pressure data are best represented as a movie, showing the changing location and pressure pattern through stance phase. However, for printed material it is typically represented as a figure that shows the peak pressure at each location through the entire stance phase for a single step. The path of the center of pressure (COP) can be overlaid on the picture, representing the location of the center of all pressure at each point in time, from initial contact to foot-off. Holmes et al. (1991) and Orlin and McPoil (2000) provide good references for established foot-pressure products and data-collection techniques.

24

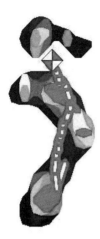
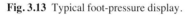
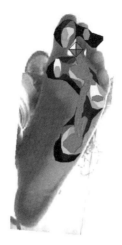

Fig. 3.13 Typical foot-pressure display.

Fig. 3.14 Enhanced foot-pressure display, overlaid on a static photo of the individual's foot.

ENERGY EXPENDITURE

The volume of oxygen uptake (VO_2) during respiration is a useful indicator of energy efficiency during gait. Analysis of energy expenditure is typically performed using portable telemetry system incorporating a mask worn around the face (Fig. 3.15). Data are typically reported as the volume of oxygen used per unit time (oxygen consumption) or oxygen used per unit distance (oxygen cost). Oxygen cost is affected by a subject's velocity, while oxygen consumption is independent of velocity. Oxygen utilization analysis does not give any information regarding mechanics, risk for injury, or quality of gait, as the other data types mentioned here provide. However, oxygen utilization measurements provide information regarding the efficiency of gait, which none of the other gait-analysis indices described provide directly. Oxygen utilization is frequently used as a functional outcome measure. For example, solid AFOs have been shown to decrease energy expenditure during gait in children with spastic cerebral palsy (Maltais et al. 2001) and myelomeningocoele (Duffy et al. 2000).

Measuring outcomes

Revisiting the assessment using the above criteria is one way of assessing any change. However, each of the assessments described are subject to some degree of measurement error because of limitations in repeatability and inter-observer differences. Therefore it can be difficult to measure accurately any benefit from using orthoses; and sometimes, as in the case of progressive conditions, no change is actually a good outcome.

PROFESSIONALLY ASSESSED INSTRUMENTS

A number of standardised assessment methods have been developed in an effort to reduce measurement error and variation between assessments. These instruments must have been

Fig. 3.15. Typical equipment for measuring energy expenditure including face mask and belt computer.

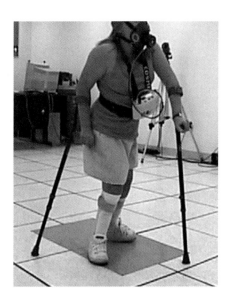

shown to be valid and reliable for their stated purpose in order to be useful. We have acknowledged already that the ordinal systems used for assessing muscle strength (MRC Scale) are crude compared to measurements made using dynamometers. The Gross Motor Function Measure (GMFM), which can be used for assessing the gross-motor abilities of children with cerebral palsy and Down syndrome, involves the child attempting a number of tasks (Russell et al. 2002). The Pediatric Evaluation of Disability Inventory (PEDI) provides a way of assessing a child's functional performance in typical daily activities such as dressing and eating (Haley et al. 1992). Similarly, the Assessment of Life Habits (LIFE-H) provides a means for evaluating the effects of any impairment on children's activities and participation (Fougeyrollas et al. 2003)

FAMILY-ASSESSED INSTRUMENTS
Patient-assessed outcomes are increasingly used with adults; to a lesser extent, they are also used to evaluate children's health care. Family-assessed instruments for use in paediatric orthopaedics were recently reviewed by a group in Canada (Furlong et al. 2005). For any particular application, clinicians can choose from a battery of instruments such as the Activities Scale for Kids, which is a generic measure of physical functioning in the community for children between 5 and 15 years old (Young et al. 2000). There are several condition-specific measures, for instance for assessing the severity of foot problems associated with juvenile chronic arthritis (Andre et al. 2004), or quality of life associated with scoliosis (Feise et al. 2005). These instruments are intended to address the more specific issues associated with those conditions and specifically from the child and family's perspective.

References

Andre M, Hagelberg S, Stenstrom CH (2004) The juvenile arthritis foot disability index: development and evaluation of measurement properties. *J Rheumatol* **31**: 2488–93.

Brunnekreef JJ, van Uden CJ, van Mooresel S, Kooloos JG (2005) Reliability of videotaped observational gait analysis in patients with orthopedic impairments. *BMC Musculoskel Disord* **17**: 17.

Condie DN, Stewart CPU (1997) The orthotic supply process. In: Condie DN, Stewart CPU, Jain AS, Rowley DI, Dolan MJ, eds. *Orthotics*. Distance Learning Section, Dept of Orthopaedic and Trauma Surgery, University of Dundee.

Duffy CM, Graham HK, Cosgrove AP. (2000) The influence of ankle–foot orthoses on gait and energy expenditure in spina bifida. *J Pediatr Orthop* **20**: 356–61.

Feise RJ, Donaldson S, Crowther ER, Menke JM, Wright JG (2005) Construction and validation of the scoliosis quality of life index in adolescent idiopathic scoliosis. *Spine* **30**: 1310–15.

Fougeyrollas P, Noreau L, Lepage C (2003) *Assessment of Life Habits (LIFE-H for Children 1.0) Adapted for Children 5–13 Years. Short and Long Forms*. Lac-Saint-Charles, Quebec: INDCP.

Furlong W, Barr RD, Feeny D, Yandow S (2005) Patient-focused measures of functional health status and health-related quality of life in pediatric orthopedics: a case study in measurement selection. *Health Qual Life Outcomes* **3**: 3.

Gage J (2004) *The Treatment of Gait Problems in Cerebral Palsy*. London: Mac Keith Press.

Holmes GB Jr, Timmerman L, Willits NH (1991) Practical considerations for the use of the pedobarograph. *Foot Ankle* **12**: 105–8.

Haley SM, Coster WJ, Ludlow LH, Haltiwanger JT, Andrellos PJ (1992) *Pediatric Evaluation of Disability Inventory: Development, Standardization, and Administration Manual, Version 1.0*. Boston, MA: Trustees of Boston University, Health and Disability Research Institute.

King SM, Rosenbaum PL, King GA (1996) Parents' perceptions of development and validation of a measured of processes. *Dev Med Child Neurol* **38**: 757–72.

Krebs DE, Edelstein JE, Fishman S (1985) Reliability of observational kinematic gait analysis. *Phys Ther* **65**: 1027–33.

Lam WK, Leong JC, Li YH, Hu Y, Lu WW (2005) Biomechanical and electromyographic evaluation of ankle foot orthosis and dynamic ankle foot orthosis in spastic cerebral palsy. *Gait Posture* **22**: 189–97.

Maltais D, Bar-Or O, Galea V, Pierrynowski M. (2001) Use of orthoses lowers the O_2 cost of walking in children with spastic cerebral palsy. *Med Sci Sports Exerc* **33**: 320–5.

Orlin M, McPoil T (2000) Plantar pressure assessment. *Phys Ther* **80**: 399–409.

Park BK, Song HR, Vankoski SJ, Moore CA, Dias LS. (1997) Gait electromyography in children with myelomeningocele at the sacral level. *Arch Phys Med Rehabil* **78**: 471–5.

Perry J (1992) *Gait Analysis: Normal and Pathological Function*. Thorofare, NJ: Slack.

Rosenbaum PL, King SM, Cadman DT (1992) Measuring processes of caregiving to physically disabled children and their families. I: Identifying relevant components of care. *Dev Med Child Neurol* **34**: 103–14.

Russell D, Rosenbaum P, Avery L, Lane M (2002) *Gross Motor Function Measure (GMFM-66 & GMFM-88) Users' Manual*. London: Mac Keith Press.

Sutherland D, Olshen R, Biden E, Wyatt M (1988) *The Development of Mature Walking*. London: Mac Keith Press.

Young NL, Williams JI, Yoshida KK, Wright JG (2000) Measurement properties of the Activities Scale for Kids. *J Clin Epidemiol* **53**: 125-37.

4
MATERIALS, COMPONENTS AND FABRICATION

Christopher Morris

Traditionally orthoses were constructed from metal and leather, rendering them heavy and unsightly; however, contemporary orthoses made with plastics can be lightweight and hidden more easily under clothing. This chapter outlines the materials commonly used to fabricate orthoses, including some components that are commercially available; first there is consideration of the fabrication process.

Overview of fabrication

Once the decision has been taken about which orthosis is to be made, the manufacturing process begins with recording key measurements including circumferences, widths and lengths and also often making a cast model of the relevant part of the body. Details of all the necessary measurements are crucial to ensure the successful fit of any orthosis; as far as possible, the cast should represent the intended posture in the orthosis (Fig. 4.1). The skills involved in taking good casts are a mixture of technique and practice, and there is rarely a right or wrong way to achieve the end result; orthotists develop various methods, and much can be learnt from visiting different centres to glean ideas. The negative cast is subsequently

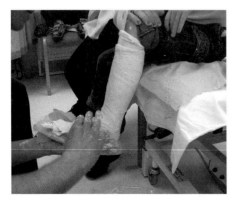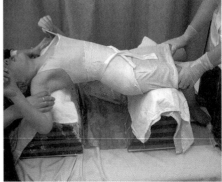

Fig. 4.1 The taking of accurate plaster casts provides the best chance of producing well-fitting orthoses, there are a variety of techniques and rarely any right or wrong method.

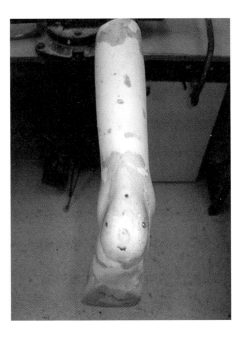

Fig. 4.2 The positive cast model is modified and smoothed in preparation for moulding; coloured dye has been added to distinguish the added plaster from the original cast.

filled and discarded, leaving the positive model which is used in the fabrication process (Fig. 4.2).

As it is rare for orthotists to fabricate the entire orthosis themselves, the specification for the orthosis and measurements must then be communicated to the technician. It is vital that there is a shared understanding of what is to be produced; some workshops have manuals with basic orthotic designs that can be modified and have quality-assurance procedures. In some workshops one technician will fabricate the entire orthosis, whilst in other centres there is a production line in which technicians specialize in key parts of the process such as metal, plastic or leatherwork. Orthotic organizations vary in size; some operate central fabrication hubs, with several orthotists operating often far away in other cities, whilst other operations may be much smaller and localized. In principle, although the author's preference is to have a local workshop so that all aspects of construction can be monitored, both systems can be efficient, provided that the manufacturing process is well managed. What is very important for children is that any orthosis does not take long to make (since children grow), and that if any repair is necessary the child is without the orthosis for the minimum time (as the child's activities may be limited or the treatment effect reduced). One advantage of having a workshop integral to the clinic is that repairs and alterations can often be done on the same day.

The parts of the orthosis are made and assembled, together with any components and fastenings. When making complex orthoses a trial fitting stage before the orthosis is finished can be useful, to check the that fit is correct. However, whenever possible – again to avoid any unnecessary delay – the aim should usually be to fit and supply the orthosis at the appointment immediately following the taking of the measurements. This is why it is so important to record and communicate the measurements, and to pay close attention to every detail; then, with basic workshop facilities available close to the clinic, any small modifications to the new orthosis can be made at the time of supply.

Materials

PLASTICS

A variety of plastics have become available since the 1960s; for our purposes these can be broadly classified into two groups, those that are formable at low temperatures and those that require higher temperatures to make them pliable. So-called low-temperature thermoplastics can be moulded directly to the body after softening in hot water; high-temperature thermoplastics, often heated to 200°C. are moulded to plaster models of the child's body. Low-temperature thermoplastics are not as strong and are used for upper-limb applications or for making night-time and postoperative orthoses. The commonest high-temperature plastic used in orthotics is polypropylene; polythene is also sometimes used. To confuse matters there are different grades of each plastic depending on the molecular structure and what compounds have been added. For the general reader it is enough to know that the sheets come in different thicknesses and colours; child-friendly patterns can also be added to the sheets when they are hot, before moulding takes place.

In a process called 'drape-forming', the molten sheets are laid over the casts and the ends welded together, while any excess material is trimmed and the plastic cools and forms into the shape of the cast. To achieve a closer-fitting orthosis, it is possible to mould the plastic sheet over a tube connected to a vacuum pump (Fig. 4.3); the pump is turned on to evacuate the air once the hot plastic is sealed around the cast and tube, and the pressure differential is maintained until the plastic has cooled. Any components such as side members for knee–ankle–foot orthoses (KAFOs), ankle hinges or padding can be added to the cast prior to moulding so that they are part of the moulded shell (Fig. 4.4). The shell is then trimmed off from the cast when it is cool and cut and ground down to the required shape

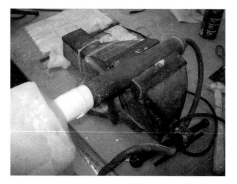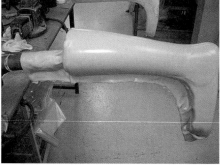

Fig. 4.3 The stem of the cast is inserted into a tube connected to an air compressor, once the plastic is sealed over the cast and tube, the air is extracted to create a vacuum.

30

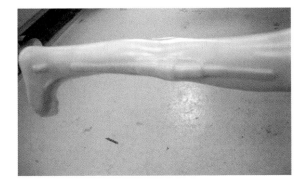

Fig. 4.4 Polypropylene moulded over orthotic knee and ankle hinges to fabricate a KAFO.

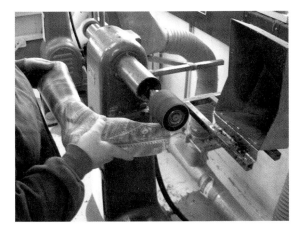

Fig. 4.5 The plastic shell is trimmed and ground to shape and the edges polished to remove any notches.

(Fig. 4.5). One great advantage of using plastics, and polypropylene in particular, is that small areas can be locally heated and adjusted to create more or less space at any time.

FOAMS AND RUBBERS

There are two types of foam material used in orthotics: those with an open cell-structure, which tend to compress easily, and closed-cell foams which tend to be more resilient. The density of the foam (low, medium or high) is often used to describe its properties. Thin (3–5mm) layers of polyurethane foam are useful for padding over bony prominences inside plastic orthoses. Thicker sheets of ethylene vinyl acetate (EVA) foams are used to make foot orthoses by vacuum moulding the material when hot inside a sealable metal box with a flexible membrane (Fig. 4.6).

METALS

Metals offer greater stiffness and strength than plastics; the disadvantage is that they are usually heavier. As metals offer high resistance to bending they are the most appropriate material for the side members of KAFOs and hip–knee–ankle–foot orthoses (HKAFOs). The two metals most commonly used are steel and aluminium; steel is by far the stronger, but

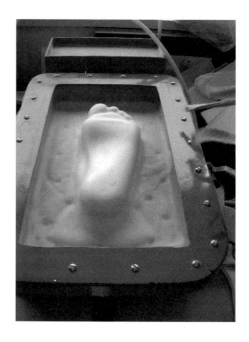

Fig. 4.6 Extracting air from a box covered by a flexible diaphragm creates a 'vacuum' for moulding polypropylene or EVA foot orthoses.

aluminium is lighter and more ductile and easy to form. Most steel used in orthotics is treated to create a 'stainless' outer skin. Metal side members are bought as modular components, cut to length and then cold-formed for the individual child (Fig. 4.7). The metal is then drilled and tapped to enable the plastic section to be attached with screws, so that small changes in length can be accommodated. Metal rivets are often used to secure the straps to metal, leather or plastic orthoses or to attach components together permanently.

LEATHERS

Leathers are natural materials, and are therefore variable in terms of their properties; however, there are certain classes of leather that are appropriate for key orthotic applications. For example, chamois leather provides a suitably thin lining material to be used next to the skin inside plastic orthoses; sheepskin is useful for protecting skin and providing warmth. More durable calf or chrome leathers are used to reinforce Velcro straps or cover metal substructures. Leathers are often initially glued and then either hand- or machine-stitched.

FABRICS

Natural cotton or synthetic (often nylon or elastic) fabrics are used to fabricate orthoses such as in wraparound arm or knee gaiters, or wrist–hand orthoses. One of the most common fabric materials is Velcro, used for the fastening on most orthoses. There has been interest in using Lycra or similar fabrics to make orthoses, particularly for the upper limb.

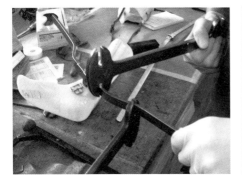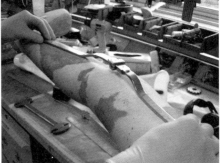

Fig. 4.7 Cold forming metal to shape side members for a KAFO.

COMPOSITES

Plaster of Paris and synthetic casting materials are examples of composite materials made up of fibres that are held in a fixed position as the matrix material sets. Whilst it is possible to construct orthoses by laminating fibre sheets with epoxy resins, as is done routinely when making prosthetic sockets, these methods are rarely employed in paediatric orthotics. Composite materials enable one to make extremely light devices and to tailor the properties of strength and flexibility to different parts of the shell of an orthosis. However, the methods are considerably more expensive than using plastics and cannot easily be adjusted as the child grows or if their condition changes.

Components

ORTHOTIC HINGES

Orthoses are often used to stabilize joints of the body, and whilst sometimes the orthosis will immobilize the joint, at other times movement can be facilitating by incorporating an orthotic hinge. The range of motion available from the hinge may be unrestricted, controlled within a limited range, or perhaps locked for some activity such as walking and unlocked at other times such as when sitting. Further examples of various hinges can be found in the chapters on upper- and lower-limb orthoses.

REINFORCEMENTS

Composite (carbon fibre) components can be used to reinforce specific areas in plastic orthoses for example to make the ankle area more rigid. Localized stiffening of an orthosis can also be achieved at any area by simply moulding over a rib of foam material as some of the increased resistance to bending is gained by creating a corrugation in the plastic.

5
UPPER-LIMB ORTHOSES

Nicole Parent-Weiss

Upper-limb orthoses do not usually have to withstand the high forces generated during weight-bearing, and so can usually be fabricated using lighter materials that are not as stiff or strong as those used in the lower limb. Plastics that can be moulded at a temperature low enough to be applied directly onto the body are useful because they can be easily adjusted and accommodate changes in the clinical picture. This adaptability is a great advantage when one considers the intricacies of managing the hand and fingers in particular. However, there are also times when it will be more suitable to use orthoses made from high-temperature thermoplastics, such as polypropylene and polyethylene, moulded to a plaster model of the child's arm.

Hand orthoses (HdOs)
Hand orthoses control one or more of the fingers and sometimes the thumb. They do not cover or attempt to control the wrist and are commonly fabricated out of a low-temperature plastic for a temporary or interim goal. We use the acronym HdO to distinguish hand orthoses from hip orthoses.

HDOS TO IMPROVE FUNCTION
The functional position of the hand is 45° metacarpophalangeal (MCP) flexion and 15° interphalangeal (IP) flexion. The thumb is positioned in abduction to facilitate thumb-to-index finger-pad opposition (Fig. 5.1). A plastic HdO can be moulded to limit the range of extension at MCP joints and trimmed proximal to the MCP joints in the palm to permit full flexion and grasping (Fig. 5.2). This design is used to compensate for intrinsic muscle weakness when MCP hyperextension can impede dexterity. With MCP hyperextension

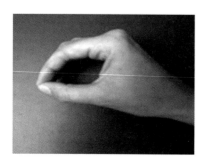

Fig. 5.1 Thumb abduction and opposition position – index finger and thumb contact.

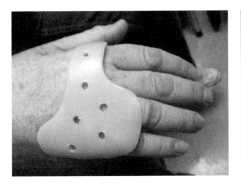
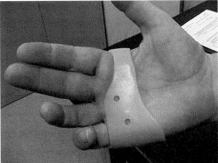

Fig. 5.2 HdO designed to limit MCP extension.

prevented, the hand is maintained in a more functional position. Hand orthoses may also include static attachments such as clips for writing or holding utensils when the ability to grasp has been lost.

Neoprene and elastic fabric HdOs are also used to place the hand in a position of function. Fabric HdOs generate heat over the joints which can be useful for therapeutic joint mobilization. Although ineffective in maintaining a palmar arch due to the flexibility of the material, fabric hand orthoses can prevent thumb adduction ('palm in hand') and maintain the thumb in a functional position. HdOs may also be used to maintain the thumb interphalangeal (IP) joint in extension if the orthosis is of sufficient length.

HdOs to Prevent or Correct Deformity

HdOs designed to immobilize the hand and fingers can be used to decrease pain or prevent joint contractures. Immobilization of the interphalangeal (IP) joints is achieved using a three-point force which applies a dorsal corrective force to promote extension, or conversely a palmar corrective force to promote flexion. This is commonly done using a prefabricated ring design.

The carpo–metacarpal (CMC) joints can be immobilized in an orthosis that contains the CMC joint and the metacarpo–phalangeal (MCP) joint, as well as the interphalangeal (IP)

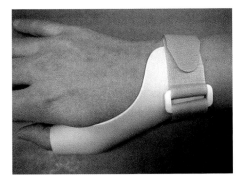

Fig. 5.3 Radially based thumb-abduction orthosis – 'gamekeeper orthosis'.

35

joint of the thumb. The orthosis extends over the radial side of the base of the palm both on the palmar and dorsal surface. A Velcro strap extends from the HdO medially, across the lateral aspect of the palm. The thumb is positioned in abduction and in opposition to the middle and index fingers (Fig. 5.3).

The loss of power in the intrinsic muscles in the hand, sometimes called *intrinsic minus*, predisposes the hand to MCP hyperextension combined with flexion of the IP joints. In these circumstances the HdO will hold the MCPs in 90° of flexion and the interphalangeal joints in full extension. This prevents contracture of the lumbricals and interosseous hand muscles which actively flex the MCP and extend the IP joints.

HdOs that include elastics or springs can generate active forces for stretching. These are used in therapeutic regimens to increase the range of extension in the IP joint of the fingers or thumb. Elastic finger loops can also be attached to a glove to increase the range of IP joint flexion.

Wrist–hand orthoses (WHOs)
WHOs extend from any level distal to the elbow and include part or all of the hand. The distal trimline of a WHO varies according to the clinical objective and may include controlling the fingers and thumb using the principles described in the previous section. The functional position of the wrist is 15°–20° wrist extension, slight ulnar deviation, 45° MCP flexion and 15° IP flexion. When included, as with HdOs, the thumb is positioned in abduction and opposition to the middle and index fingers as in Figure 5.1.

WHOs to Improve Function
WHOs designed to maintain the wrist in a functionally extended position may either be static or incorporate components under tension to generate active forces. For instance a dorsal-based forearm component with spring-assisted finger loops attached allows active finger flexion to assist weak or absent extension motion. Static orthoses may either be circumferential or include only dorsal or ventral plastic sections that are fastened with Velcro straps and the latter are more commonly used because of their low profile. The thumb may or may not be included. These WHOs can be moulded directly onto the child's arm but are often made using a plaster model (Fig. 5.4). Adjustments are made to accommodate bony prominences such as the ulnar styloid process, which can be susceptible to excessive pressure and rubbing. Care should also be taken during casting and fabrication to maintain the contour of the palmar arch.

Flexor hinge (tenodesis or wrist-driven) WHOs apply the principles of *functional tenodesis*. This includes finger flexion (functional prehension) elicited by active or assisted wrist extension and finger extension (functional release) elicited by active or gravity assisted wrist flexion. Functionally, when the wrist is actively or passively extended, the fingers will flex passively. This passive flexion can be used to substitute for functional grasp. When the wrist is actively or passively flexed, with gravity, the fingers passively extend and can be used to substitute for functional release. This orthosis is commonly used with a quadriplegic patient with muscular innervation to at least the C6 level. The orthosis can also be modified slightly to transform it into a ratchet WHO which includes the use of a ratchet

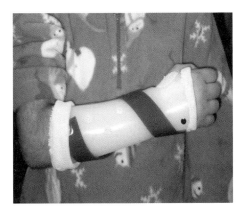

Fig. 5.4 Custom-moulded polyethylene WHO.

or incrementally locking mechanism to position the wrist in a functional position, allow completion of the task, then with activation of a quick release – reposition the wrist in neutral or wrist flexion. A ratchet orthosis may be more appropriate for a quadriplegic patient with innervation to only the C5 level.

Prefabricated WHOs are widely available with sizes that appropriately accommodate the size of the child's arm (Fig. 5.5). They are generally made of canvas, elastic or neoprene materials. The distal trim line should not extend past the distal palmar crease to allow unrestricted MCP flexion. Versions with a thumb-spica extending to the IP joint are available. If thumb immobilization is not required the thumb opening should be circular and not hinder the thenar eminence or movement of the thumb. Post-fracture care is commonly

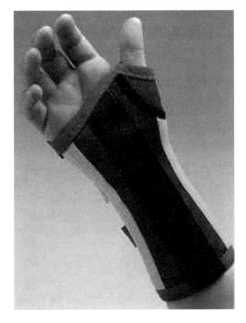

Fig. 5.5 Prefabricated WHO.

a diagnosis that requires a prefabricated WHO to prevent reinjury and protect weak muscles after immobilization or surgery.

WHOs to Prevent or Correct Deformity

Resting WHOs moulded along the ventral surface of the forearm and hand may be used to maintain range of motion in the wrist and fingers; they are sometimes referred to as 'paddle' orthoses because of their clumsy shape. Resting WHOs can be fabricated with or without a thumb–spica extension. Minor correction can be incorporated in the fabrication process, (although these orthoses are more commonly used to maintain rather than to increase range of motion) in order to be tolerable to wear (Fig. 5.6). Fastening straps should keep the hand and wrist well positioned in orthosis. One strap should always be located directly over the wrist joint, to prevent wrist flexion, as well as maintaining firm contact in the palmar arch and proximal forearm to complete a three-point force system. Holding the limb securely in the orthosis decreases the chances of compromising skin integrity.

Resting WHOs are usually used at night; though they may be worn for longer if the orthosis does not limit the child's activities. Most WHOs only extend to the mid-forearm; but in exceptional circumstances, such as post-fracture treatment of the forearm, the orthosis may be extended more proximally towards the elbow. Some control of forearm rotation can be achieved by actually encompassing the epicondyles of the elbow joint in the orthosis (Fig. 5.7), thereby limiting supination and pronation. Limiting forearm rotation may be necessary after forearm fracture.

In addition to the static designs a hinge can be incorporated at the wrist. Static progressive stretching regimens utilize a WHO incorporating a hinge that allows the joint position to be changed in small static increments. This may be achieved using either a 'worm-gear' screw design that allows continuous gradual adjustment, or a 'step-lock' design that allows a certain number of degrees between each locking position.

Elbow orthosis (EO)

The small size of the humerus and the forearm in children generally necessitates custom fabrication for most clinical situations. EOs are designed either with a solid, non-articulating elbow or may include an articulating orthotic hinge. EOs that incorporate a hinge may allow,

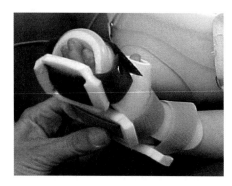

Fig. 5.6 Resting WHO.

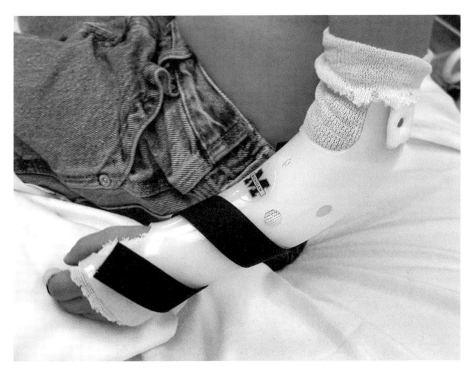

Fig. 5.7 Modified Münster-design WHO – plastic extended over epicondyles.

assist or restrict elbow joint motion as required. The orthotic elbow hinge should be aligned close to the axis defined by the medial and lateral epicondyles.

EOS TO IMPROVE FUNCTION

Elbow orthoses may enable function dependent on the injury or clinical situation. A forearm cuff connected to a humeral cuff with a simple hinge will provide medial–lateral stability whilst allowing flexion–extension motion. The articulation may allow the full range of motion, or incorporate some form of motion limitation to restrict the available range of flexion and extension between a set range of motion (i.e. 30°–90°). They can also be locked to function as a solid elbow in the early stages of healing or post-injury. This may be appropriate following elbow dislocation when full elbow extension places the elbow in a vulnerable position for re-dislocation. The wrist and hand may not necessarily be included in the orthosis, although their inclusion may help to secure the orthosis onto the arm. Extension of the distal component to include the wrist and hand facilitates control of forearm rotation. The forearm is often left in full supination to protect injury to medial elbow ligamentous structures or status post radial head dislocations (Fig. 5.8). The forearm may alternatively be left in fully pronated to protect against lateral elbow ligamentous injury or disruption.

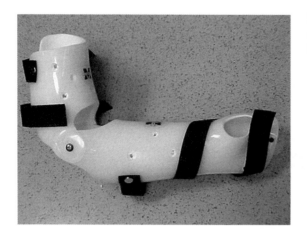

Fig. 5.8 Custom EO positioned in neutral forearm rotation (to prevent pronation).

EOS TO PREVENT OR CORRECT DEFORMITY

The effective use of static progressive stretching (SPS) orthoses for treating elbow contractures in *adults* has been documented in the literature (Green and McCoy 1979, Bonutti et al. 1994, O'Driscoll et al. 1996). The principles can, however, also be adapted for children. SPS utilizes the principle of *stress relaxation*, in which the amount of force required to maintain tissue at a given length decreases over time. The orthosis applies a corrective force slightly exceeding the elastic limit of the shortened tissues and results in relaxation and lengthening of the tissues over time. The slack is taken up gradually to increase the range of joint motion.

The appropriate EO design will include custom-moulded polyethylene humeral and forearm components lined with softer material, connected with a fixed bar or hinge, and fastenings. To ensure that the pressure resulting from the corrective force is distributed evenly across the plastic anterior parts, the openings for the humeral and forearm cuff are usually positioned posteriorly. An olecranon pad then provides the third point of the three-point force system (Fig. 5.9).

Whilst there are reasonable lengths of leverage to manage elbow-flexion contractures, controlling forearm rotation presents a more difficult challenge. One way to overcome the difficulty of simulating the longitudinal anatomical axis is to use overlapping components which include the entire forearm from the radial head to the ulnar head and includes the wrist and hand (Fig. 5.10). An orthotic hinge must be included at the elbow with extension of the orthosis over the humerus to isolate forearm rotation motion. The orthotic elbow hinge may either be solid, or have limited or free motion, or include a static progressive articulation (Gelinas et al. 2000).

EOs to prevent or correct deformity may alternatively incorporate elastic, compressed gas pistons or spring components that generate active forces. These orthoses aim to increase the range of joint motion utilizing the theory of *creep*, which is 'the continual elongation of tissue over time with the application of a constant load' (Richard et al. 1995).

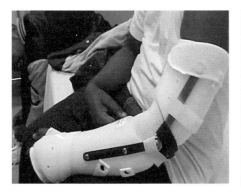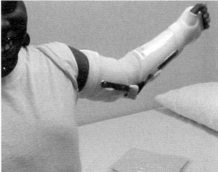

Fig. 5.9 Hinged static progressive elbow-extension orthosis.

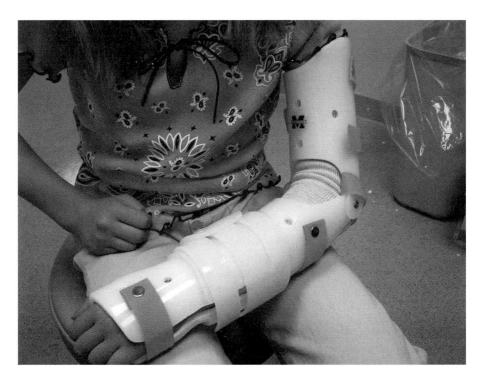

Fig. 5.10 Static progressive forearm-rotation orthosis.

When the aim of the orthosis is to increase the range of flexion, the efficacy of any hinged orthosis will become limited when the plastic of the humeral section comes in contact with the plastic of the forearm section. A second stage of design may be a shoulder-based hyperflexion EO (Fig. 5.11a, b). The forearm cuff is threaded through a loop attached to the

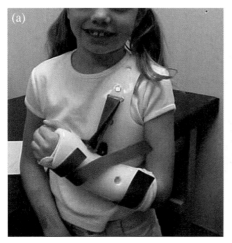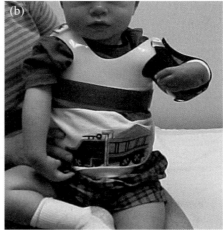

Fig. 5.11 (a) Unilateral shoulder-based flexion sling orthosis (static progressive). (b) Bilateral shoulder-based flexion sling orthosis (static progressive).

most superior aspect of the shoulder ring and the arm is positioned at a submaximal position of stretch for a longer duration of approximately 2–3 hours.

Humeral orthoses
Humeral orthoses encompass the upper arm only and are primarily used to treat fractures. They are generally custom-moulded using a circumferential polythene shell that extends to the acromian process of the shoulder. This is held securely with a thoracic strap across the contralateral shoulder. A humeral orthosis must be easily adjustable to allow for changes in volume due to oedema and swelling. The distal trim lines must be adjusted to allow full elbow flexion as joint motion will stimulate osteogenesis and bone healing. This method of immobilization attempts to prevent secondary complications associated with prolonged immobilization primarily contracture. However, the main limitation in using humeral orthoses with children, as with most acute fracture orthoses, is compliance. More often humeral designs are used with children after the healing process is well under way. The goal of protection and prevention of reinjury of the humerus is therefore more common.

Shoulder–elbow–wrist–hand–orthosis (SEWHO)
SEWHOs can exert control over shoulder flexion–extension, internal–external rotation and abduction–adduction. The torso is generally encompassed as well as the humerus to provide a biomechanical lever arm, and any orthotic shoulder hinge is located below the axilla. The use of SEWHOs to enable function in children is a rare objective; however, there are occasions when SEWHOs are used to prevent or correct deformity.

SEWHOS TO PREVENT OR CORRECT DEFORMITY

A SEWHO may be used to maintain the shoulder in a position of maximum containment where dislocation has occurred. The orthosis must be adjustable to accommodate the changes that occur, particularly when surgery is planned. This orthosis comprises a custom moulded polythene arm shell, either with a solid or articulating elbow hinge, and torso component to aid suspension. Although prefabricated designs are available, their usefulness can be limited for children of small stature.

SEWHOs also include the conventional arm sling. An addition to the sling used to treat humeral fractures is the *sling and swathe*. The swathe helps to position the shoulder in internal rotation as well as preventing abduction. Additional straps can be used to retract the shoulder for clavicle fractures.

References

Bonutti PM, Windau JE, Ables BA, Miller BG (1994) Static progressive stretch to reestablish elbow range of motion. *Clin Orthopaed* **303**: 128–34.

Gelinas JJ, Faber KJ, Patterson SD, King GJW (2000) The effectiveness of turnbuckle splinting for elbow contractures. *J Bone Joint Surg Br* **82**: 74–8.

Green DP, McCoy H (1979) Turnbuckle orthotic correction of elbow flexion contractures after acute injuries. *J Bone Joint Surg Am* **61**: 1092–5.

O'Driscoll SW, Shankland SW, Beaton D (1996) Patient adjusted static elbow splints for elbow contractures: a preliminary report. *J Shoulder Elbow Surg* **5**: suppl. 73.

Richard R, Shanesy CP 3rd, Miller SF (1995) Dynamic versus static splints: a prospective case for sustained stress. *J Burn Care Rehabil* **16**: 284–7.

6
LOWER-LIMB ORTHOSES

Christopher Morris

This chapter describes the most common lower-limb orthoses used for children. The orthoses are described in order, beginning with those applied most distally and then progressing proximally. In many cases details from the preceding sections will be relevant to subsequent parts when the orthosis also includes the distal segment. For instance knee–ankle–foot orthoses may include features described in the section on ankle–foot orthoses, and likewise ankle–foot orthoses may incorporate features described in the section on foot orthoses. Orthoses which have the primary aim of improving a child's physical functioning are listed separately from those which have the primary goal of preventing or correcting deformity.

Foot orthoses (FOs)

FOs to Improve Function

Insoles, heel pads – prefabricated and flat inlays
The simplest FO consists of a flat laminated card or leather base on which are fixed specially shaped pads of foam rubber, most commonly to support the arches of the foot. The base can be the full length of the shoe insole, or trimmed to finish proximal to the metatarsal heads so as not to fill up the forepart unnecessarily. The pads may be intended to support the medial arch, or to cushion or relieve pressure from a painful area of the plantar surface of the foot such as the metatarsal heads or heel. Padding can be used in the forepart of the shoe to compensate for a shoe-size discrepancy, allowing a child to wear a pair of shoes the same size. Heel elevators inside the shoe can compensate for leg-length discrepancies (LLDs) of up to 15 mm. Heel pads made from rubber with viscoelastic properties can be used to cushion impact forces during walking and running. Prefabricated contoured insoles designed to support the medial arch are also available (Fig. 6.1).

Moulded insoles
Insoles that are made from materials moulded over a modified plaster model of the foot can provide closer control than flat or prefabricated insoles and more effectively redistribute plantar pressure. An impression or cast of the child's foot is required, and this shape can be modified in the workshop to suit the purpose of the insole. Insoles can be made from a foam plastic material, ethylene vinyl acetate (EVA; Fig. 6.2), although there are in fact a various densities of the material available with different properties. EVA insoles are generally

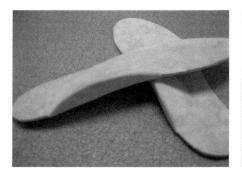

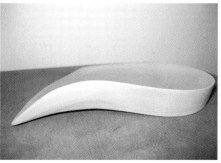

Fig. 6.1 Simple inlays consist of pre-shaped sponge rubber pads that are stuck to leather or card bases and covered with leather.

Fig. 6.2 EVA insoles with additional medial heel wedging.

bulkier than other insoles and provide less control than more rigid plastic insoles; they are easily tolerated, however, as they are softer and more flexible, and can offer some shock absorption.

FOs made from plastics such as polypropylene are similarly custom-moulded to a plaster model of the child's foot (Fig. 6.3). The quality of detail and position in the negative impression is of premier importance and various techniques have been proposed. During casting, pressure can be applied under the sustentaculum tali and peroneal notch to stabilize the calcaneus and hindfoot. The area around the navicular and base of the fifth metatarsal may also be marked and accentuated to avoid excessive pressure on these bony prominences. Greater control of the subtalar and midtarsal joints is achieved with increasing depth of the orthosis with varying amounts of mediolateral flanges and heel cupping. The design was first published by Campbell and Inman (1971) and labelled the UC-BL (University of California Biomechanics Laboratory) heel insert. Some orthotists prefer using thinner more flexible plastics to make circumferential orthoses that enclose the whole foot.

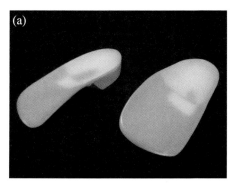
(a)

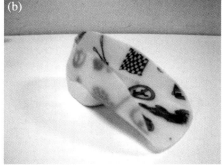
(b)

Fig. 6.3 (a) Polypropylene foot orthosis and (b) UC-BL heel cup.

Wedging can be added to the base of any of these shells to tilt the hind- or forefoot during weight-bearing. Similarly, increasing the width of the base of the insole can enhance stability. The addition of wedges and stabilizers are often referred to as 'posting' the orthosis. The aim is to align the hindfoot with the lower leg, the hindfoot with the forefoot, and the foot relative to the floor so that the foot and ankle function optimally. The principle is that the foot functions best when the subtalar joint is in its 'neutral' position, neither inverted nor everted. Consequently these insoles are sometimes referred to as 'functional foot orthoses' and fabricated subsequent to accurate biomechanical examination and analysis. The concepts were originally detailed by Root (1971) and are well described by Anthony (1991) and Philps (1995). Simplistically, lateral forefoot wedging can often be helpful in controlling hindfoot varus, and likewise medial forefoot wedging can be helpful in controlling hindfoot valgus. As the shell is fairly rigid the base of the FO is usually trimmed proximal to the metatarsal heads so as not to restrict metatarsal–phalangeal joint motion.

Supramalleolar orthoses (SMOs)
By extending the structure of a moulded plastic FO proximally over the malleoli, all the hindfoot and ankle joints are encompassed. However, although the ankle joints are within the orthosis, the length of lever available above the ankle is relatively short and this can result in excessive pressure at the top edge of the orthosis when there is major hindfoot instability. The design is typically circumferential and the foot is totally enclosed within the orthosis (Fig. 6.4). The plastic used is usually thin and flexible which allows some small movement of the foot and orthosis to occur without excessive friction at the body orthosis interface. The SMO is occasionally referred to as a dynamic ankle–foot orthosis (DAFO); however, as stated in the introduction, the title is vague and open to misinterpretation as many other orthoses use the term 'dynamic' to mean different things. The SMO design can control coronal- or transverse-plane ankle and foot deformities, as it has a little more leverage than a submalleolar design, but it does not control plantaflexion or dorsiflexion in the sagittal plane. For this the orthosis must extend proximally to just below the knee.

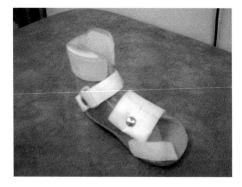

Fig. 6.4 Circumferential supramalleolar orthosis.

Footwear and footwear adaptations

The trend for health services to supply orthopaedic footwear for children with physical disabilities has declined considerably with the use of inexpensive moulded plastic foot and ankle–foot orthoses. Plastic orthoses provide greater control and are lighter, and also – because children can wear the same shoes as their peers – the social stigma of wearing 'special shoes' is avoided. However, there are occasions when providing special footwear may still be beneficial. Supportive shoes or boots may help infants with ankle–foot instability as they learn to stand and walk, especially if they are delayed in gaining coordination and balance skills. The broad base of the outsole and sturdy ankle support can be used when the foot is too small to obtain a satisfactory mould for a heel cup. However, unnecessarily heavy footwear can make gait more difficult in spite of better stability.

Children with exceptionally long or narrow feet (such as those with Marfan syndrome), or who have very wide or oedematous feet, including children who cannot fit their orthosis and foot in the shoe, will require help finding shoes. Fortunately there are a small number of shoemaking businesses that cater for this small market by making a range of footwear made on atypically sized lasts. Custom-made footwear may also be necessary to accommodate severe fixed deformities of the foot and ankle or unusual sizes. Regular shoes can be adapted to improve their usability; for instance Velcro straps can replace lace fastening to enable children with impaired dexterity to don their own footwear. Extra stiffening can be applied to reinforce the inside of the shoe. The outer sole or heel can be made wider, sometimes called 'floating out', and wedges can be added to the heel or sole to tilt the shoe to improve stability. Resilient foam cushioning can be inserted into the heel to dissipate forces generated when the heel hits the ground.

An LLD of up to 15 mm can be compensated for inside the shoe using an internal heel elevator or insole. When the LLD exceeds this height or if a shoe is too low cut to accommodate an internal shoe raise, then the additional material can be fixed to the underside of shoe. Modern orthotic materials and techniques facilitate modification of most types of ordinary shoes in an aesthetically pleasing and lightweight fashion, often inserting the raise within the original sole of the shoe. The height of the heel of the shoe, or pitch, will also influence the exact dimensions of the shoe raise. In order to avoid excessive pressure under the forefoot, material is added to both the sole and heel. However, because the added material will stiffen the shoe and restrict the heel from rising during gait, the raise is tapered off towards the toe end of the shoe to facilitate heel rise and tibial advancement (Fig. 6.5). This is sometimes called a 'rocker sole', and the principle can also be used when there is reduced or painful ankle motion during gait.

On the rare occasions when a conventional lower-limb orthosis design is preferred, the footwear usually requires some adaptation with a stirrup or socket to enable the orthosis to be attached. Straps that either retain the orthosis safely or are intended to correct foot or ankle posture may also be added. The metal and leather footwear modifications add to the overall weight of the orthosis and their absence is one of the reasons why contemporary plastic orthoses are so much lighter. The fact that the stirrups and side members can be seen outside the shoe is another aesthetic reason why contemporary plastic orthoses that fit inside the footwear are usually preferred.

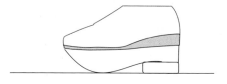

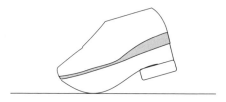

Fig. 6.5 External raises stiffen the outsole of the shoe and are therefore tapered off towards the toe end to facilitate heel rise and tibial advancement during gait. Up to 15 mm of heel raise may be accommodated inside the shoe, shown by the shaded area.

Ankle–foot orthoses (AFOs)

AFOs TO IMPROVE FUNCTION

Solid (rigid) AFOs

A plastic shell applied to the posterior calf, ankle and foot combined with strapping to retain the heel in the orthosis can be used to limit ankle plantarflexion and dorsiflexion. Extending the orthosis to just below the knee provides a long lever above the ankle, reducing the amount of force required for control (Fig. 6.6). The features described to obtain a high-quality cast and fit around the hindfoot for FOs are equally pertinent to AFOs, and additionally avoid pressure on the malleoli. Padding is frequently incorporated to dissipate pressure around these areas. Rigid AFOs can prevent plantarflexion and dorsiflexion, and also motion in the coronal and sagittal planes, most effectively when the shell extends forward around the ankle because of the distribution of material around the bending axis. Rigid or solid AFOs can also influence knee and hip motion by changing the orientation of the ground reaction force relative to the body, for instance to prevent knee hyperextension (Meadows 1984) (Fig. 6.7). The height of the heel, the pitch of the shoe, is critical when a rigid AFO is being used as this determines the inclination of the shank in the sagittal plane. This can be fine-tuned by adding or removing material until the required angle is obtained. The foot-progression angle in the transverse plane must also be noted to ensure that the calf section of the orthosis is trimmed correctly to avoid rubbing on the anterior crest of the tibia.

Control of valgus or varus tendency may be further enhanced using various straps or within the orthosis (Fig. 6.8). Some orthotists first make leather bootees to provide ankle control, and then the AFO is moulded to accommodate this; or in a similar way the orthotist may first make a plastic or leather SMO and then mould an AFO over the top. These hybrid designs provide maximum control of the foot and ankle in all planes but are generally more

Fig. 6.6 Rigid AFO.

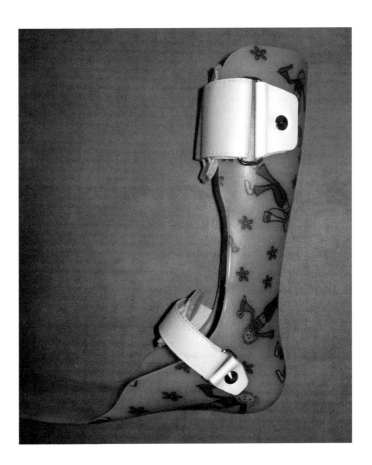

bulky and expensive. The posture of the foot relative to the ground, inside the orthosis, can be accommodated using wedging of the lateral or medial forefoot as explained in the section on foot orthoses. Extra wedging can also be added to the orthosis alter the line of action of the ground reaction force on more proximal joints and any fixed equinus can be accommodated (Fig. 6.9). It is possible to incorporate a prosthetic foot into an AFO and thereby accommodate any LLD as well as controlling the ankle and foot posture (Fig. 6.10).

When the primary goal of the orthosis is to prevent crouching as a result of excessive ankle dorsiflexion the orthosis will try to bring the ground reaction force anterior to the knee and apply force to the anterior shin. Rigidity of the ankle and footplate is vital for this design of orthosis; and a complete range of knee extension and forward-pointing foot-progression angle of the limb is critical for its success. During stance the origin of the ground reaction force moves rapidly to the distal end of the footplate of the orthosis creating an extension moment about the knee joint (Fig. 6.11). This may be optimally achieved when the ankle is fixed in slight plantarflexion providing the user has sufficient proximal muscle control to compensate for the posture this imposes. If the foot is excessively externally

49

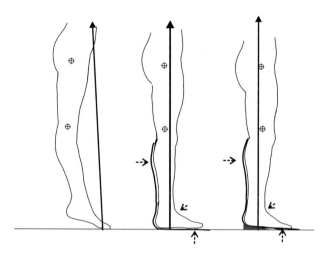

Fig. 6.7 AFOs can influence the posture of proximal joints during stance phase, preventing knee hyperextension and encouraging hip extension by altering the line of action of the ground reaction force posterior to the knee and hip joints. This may be further enhanced after appropriate 'tuning' with a heel raise.

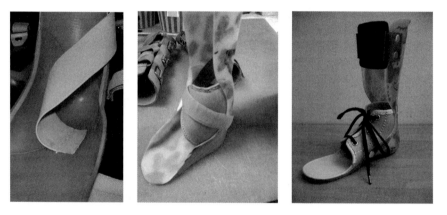

Fig. 6.8 Various corrective strapping options can enhance control of subtalar and midtarsal joint motion within the AFO.

rotated however, the length of the lever arm is reduced and may then be too short to achieve an adequate moment to maintain the ground reaction force anterior to the knee. The usual calf strap used in rigid AFOs is narrow and can result in excessive pressure over the shin. Extending the leverage proximally to the tibial tubercle and spreading the force over a greater area reduces the pressure at the body orthosis interface. Based on how they are put on, there are three common designs of 'anterior ground reaction orthosis' or AGR–AFO: the two-piece anterior entry, and the one-piece posterior and proximal entry designs (Fig. 6.12). Although all of the designs function in the same way children often find the two-piece design easier to put on and take off themselves.

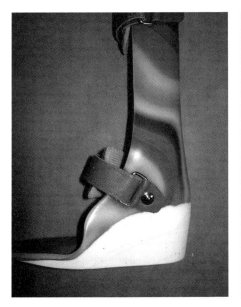

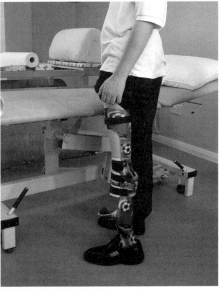

Fig. 6.9 Any fixed equinus must be accommodated and compensated for using a heel raise.

Fig. 6.10 Profound leg-length discrepancy can be accommodated by incorporating extra material and a foot prosthesis inside the AFO.

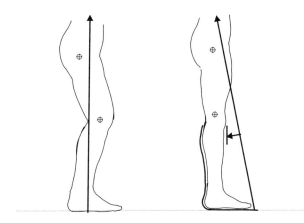

Fig. 6.11 Crouch gait is exacerbated by excessive dorsiflexion; by preventing dorsiflexion during the stance phase of gait, the origin of the ground reaction force moves rapidly forward during stance phase to the distal end of the footplate creating an extension moment about the knee joint.

If the structure of the AFO is not stiff enough to withstand the plantar and dorsiflexion moments generated during gait then the AFO may be seen to buckle at the ankle. This reduces its efficacy to influence knee and hip position. The ankle can be reinforced by simply using a thicker plastic or by moulding over a thin strip of material to create a rib or

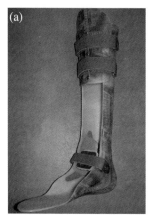 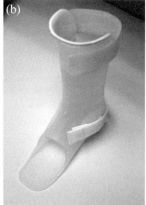 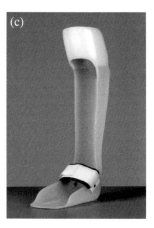

Fig. 6.12 Three designs of anterior ground reaction AFO: (a) anterior entry (two-piece), (b) posterior entry, and (c) proximal entry or Saltiel design.

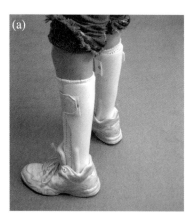 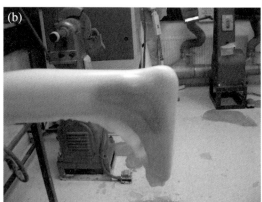

Fig. 6.13 Techniques to increase stiffness and resistance to bending in rigid AFOs: (a) ribbing, and (b) carbon fibre insert.

corrugation in the AFO at the ankle where buckling would occur (Fig. 6.13a). The ribbing has the effect of increasing the second moment or area (I-value) and stiffness, thereby increasing resistance to bending. Even greater stiffness can be achieved by moulding and including a carbon fibre–polypropylene composite insert at the ankle level. The insert component is separately heated and moulded to the positive plaster model and the AFO then moulded over the top and to which the composite insert is securely bonded in the process (Fig. 6.13b). This achieves the increased stiffness afforded by ribbing, but in addition the stiffness of the insert itself increases the stiffness of the ankle section of the orthosis. Extra layers of plastic can be laminated around the posterior part of the ankle to increase the thickness and thereby increase bending resistance. The selectively added material at the ankle prevents the side walls of the AFO bulging at the ankle and maintains the stiffness of

52

the orthosis. The footplate can likewise be stiffened by laminating an additional layer of plastic to the sole of the AFO during fabrication.

In addition to gaining mechanical advantage by extending the length of lever above the ankle, the length of footplate also influences the efficacy of the orthosis. For maximum leverage under the foot the footplate will extend forward of the full length of the shoe. However, because this can interfere with metatarsal–phalangeal joint motion in the late stance phase of gait, if the leverage is not required it may be appropriate to trim the orthosis behind the metatarsal heads. Alternatively, the plastic under the metatarsal heads can be thinned using a buffing machine to render the footplate more flexible. When the footplate is required to be rigid to maintain the ground reaction force anterior to the knee it is possible to laminate an extra sheet of plastic within the orthosis to increase the thickness and therefore resistance to bending. Modifying the shape of the footplate in the transverse plane, combined with closely fitting side walls or strapping can be used to control forefoot adduction or abduction.

Hinged AFOs

When the AFO is only designed to prevent either plantar or dorsiflexion then a hinge can be incorporated into the orthosis. The simplest way to introduce an orthotic hinge is to trim material away around the back of the ankle and heel which make the plastic more flexible at this point, often termed a *posterior leaf spring* (PLS) AFO (Fig. 6.14). The PLS–AFO is capable of limiting plantarflexion during swing phase of gait but allows dorsiflexion during stance. When there are high deforming forces the PLS–AFO may not entirely prevent plantarflexion.

There are several other ways to introduce a hinge at the ankle (Fig. 6.15). There are proprietary orthotic ankle hinges that can be introduced to the structure during the moulding process, or alternatively a two-stage moulding process can be employed and a hinge created at the level of the ankle where the two pieces of plastic overlap. These hinges usually allow free motion unless other design features are incorporated to prevent plantarflexion or dorsiflexion. For instance, a short strap can be attached posterior to the ankle joint, between the heel cup and the tibial section, to restrict tibial advancement. This provides a useful way of limiting dorsiflexion without preventing the motion altogether. When there is no requirement for the orthosis to restrict ankle motion the orthosis can be trimmed to permit free motion in the sagittal plane. Other types of ankle hinge include the adjustable ankle lock, which can be fixed in different degrees of plantarflexion or dorsiflexion, and the dorsiflexion assist which uses a concealed spring to generate an active dorsiflexing moment.

AFOs to Prevent or Correct Deformity

When the aim of an AFO is to maintain a certain position during the night, as well as or instead of during the day, there are other design issues to consider. In principle the design of the orthosis is exactly the same in terms of the corrective forces being applied, and the same AFO could be worn day and night, just changing the under-sock for hygiene. However, the high forces generated during walking and other activities are not present, and this means that less strong but lighter materials may be considered. Low-temperature plastics may be

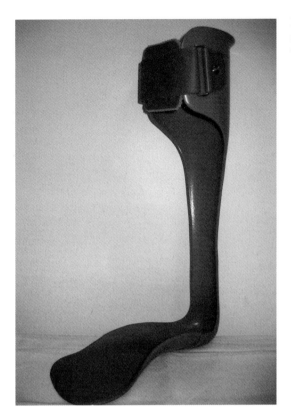

Fig. 6.14 Posterior leaf spring AFO restricts plantarflexion whilst allowing dorsiflexion.

most appropriate for infants requiring an AFO to prevent or correct a deformity as the size and posture of the child's foot will change rapidly. When considering the use of orthoses at night, a key issue is that if the orthosis is applying strong corrective forces then the child may not find it easy to sleep, and there are sometimes reports of the AFO being anywhere but on the child's leg in the morning. For this reason the orthosis is usually fabricated with the foot at a right angle (90°) to the lower leg, not allowing plantarflexion or dorsiflexion, with the hind- and forefoot similarly corrected to a midline posture that the child will tolerate.

Knee orthoses (KOs)

KOs TO IMPROVE FUNCTION
KOs do not include the ankle and foot and aim only to control the knee joint. Without any distal elements, suspension of the orthosis can be a problem, and knee orthoses are therefore prone to slipping down the leg. Fabric (commonly Lycra) KOs may be used to try and control the patella or to provide some limited support to the acutely injured knee. Greater joint instability will require more support, such as with the KOs used for sports injuries where there is damage to the cruciate ligaments.

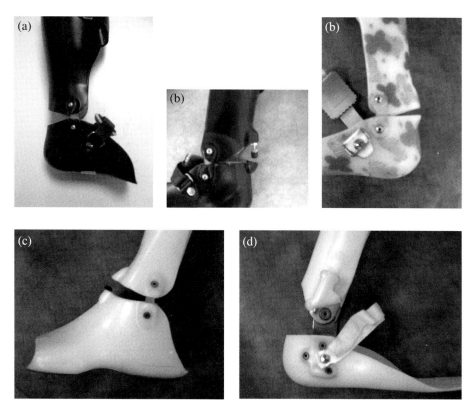

Fig. 6.15 Examples of hinged AFOs. (a) Unrestricted plantarflexion–dorsiflexion; (b) plantarflexion prevented with either solid or adjustable stop, dorsiflexion allowed; (c) dorsiflexion prevented, plantarflexion allowed; and (d) dorsiflexion assisted by spring enclosed in channel posterior to ankle joint.

KOs to Prevent or Correct Deformity

Fabric gaiters are canvas or cotton garments stiffened with metal stays, and they wrap around the leg to maintain knee extension (Fig. 6.16). They can be lined with sheepskin to avoid excessive skin pressure. It is possible to maintain knee extension using a knee orthosis only, though there can be problems with excessive pressure at both the distal and proximal edges due to the shortened leverage. Extension of the orthosis to the foot using a trough design lengthens the lever exerting a moment about the knee and hence reducing the force applied, enabling the gastrocnemius to be stretched in addition to the soft tissues around the knee joint.

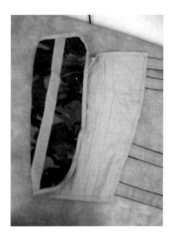

Fig. 6.16 Fabric knee gaiter, can be used to maintain knee extended during activities or in conjunction with an AFO to stretch the gastrocnemius muscle.

Knee–ankle–foot orthoses (KAFOs)

KAFOs to Improve Function

KAFOs extend from the thigh to control the knee joint in addition to controlling the ankle and foot. The thigh section may be continuous with the material of the AFO or be joined to it using metal sidebars. Two sidebars are usually required to provide the necessary rigidity for a KAFO, although occasionally for infants a lateral bar may provide sufficient support and reduce the weight and bulk of the orthosis. The sidebars may include an orthotic knee hinge depending on the need or ability of the child to bend the knee. If there is no functional knee flexion, or the orthosis will only be worn with the knee extended, then the use of an orthotic knee hinge merely adds unnecessary bulk, weight and expense to the orthosis.

When there is no indication to prevent knee flexion or extension, an orthotic knee hinge that moves freely in the sagittal plane can be used. If there is severe hyperextension of the knee at mid-stance, which cannot be controlled using an AFO to influence the ground reaction force, one design of orthotic free knee hinge called the 'posterior offset' or 'setback' knee hinge can be used (Fig. 6.17). The orthotic knee-hinge axis is positioned posterior to the knee during fabrication of the orthosis. During gait, when positioned correctly, the orthotic hinge reaches full extension before the knee and provides the necessary structural integrity for the orthosis to prevent knee hyperextension.

More commonly the KAFO is used to compensate for weak knee-extensors or instability. In these instances the orthosis is locked in extension during activity but may be unlocked during sitting. There are many proprietary brands of orthotic knee hinges used in different countries that are generally variations on common designs (Fig. 6.18). One key issue when selecting an appropriate locking knee hinge is to consider how and who is going to be responsible for locking and unlocking the mechanism. Some designs can require two hands, such as the ring-catch, and some can be unlocked with only one hand. The release bar can be positioned behind the knee, which makes it easy to simply lay the leg into the KAFO when putting the orthosis on; alternatively, the release mechanism can be fitted

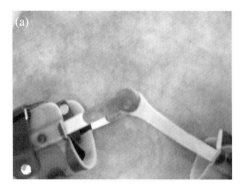

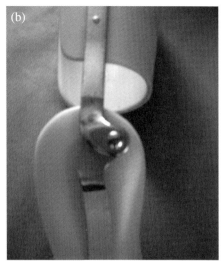

Fig. 6.17 Orthotic knee hinges with unrestricted flexion. (a) Simple hinge allows full range of flexion to full knee extension. (b) Posterior off-set (or set-back) hinge useful for preventing knee hyperextension without limiting knee flexion.

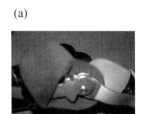

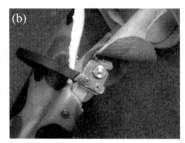

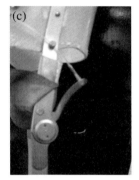

Fig. 6.18 Examples of locking orthotic knee hinges. (a) Ring lock may include enclosed springs for automatic locking in extension. (b) 'Chailey' lock is a variation of the ring-lock that additionally includes an anterior cam release mechanism which enables the joint to be unlocked one-handed at the front whilst under load. This is often useful for children with upper limb weakness as the bar is easy to reach and grasp. (c) Bale lock, can be used as two-handed trigger release, or triggers connected with anterior cable mechanism, or joined at back for one-handed posterior release.

anterior to the knee hinge, which means the leg has to be threaded through when putting the orthosis on, but is easier for the child to operate. New developments in the design of orthotic knee hinges may in the future provide orthoses that are stable during stance and flex freely at the knee during swing phase. These are only just beginning to be tested for adults, however, and are not yet available in sizes suitable for children.

Orthotic knee hinges are usually pre-set with 5° of knee flexion, but this can be modified when making the KAFO to accommodate approximately 25°–30° of fixed knee flexion. However, with increasing degrees of knee flexion, greater forces will be required to maintain the position and may not be tolerated at the body orthosis interface. The forces will be least when the knee is fully extended so this is the most desirable position in which to make the KAFO. There are several options for applying the extending force anterior to the leg. One can have a leather kneecap with straps fastening around the sidebars but it is not always desirable to apply pressure directly to the joint and patella. Therefore one can use either infrapatellar (below the knee) or suprapatellar straps (above the knee). The difficulty with these designs of knee control straps is that they are dependent on the straps being fastened to the correct tension to maintain the knee fully extended. When a child is using KAFOs on both legs, failure to get the knees equally extended will result in postural asymmetry. One way around these problems is to mould the anterior knee control mechanism in plastic and rivet it in a fixed position (Fig. 6.19). This means that whenever the KAFO is locked in extension the knee will be in the expected position. In addition to the knee-control straps or pads there will usually be straps to retain the heel in the AFO section and to secure the thigh section. The AFO section may utilize any of the hinge designs or be rigid and may be reinforced with ribbing as discussed in the preceding section.

KAFOs to Prevent or Correct Deformity

In order to stretch the gastrocnemius muscles the ankle must be dorsiflexed with simultaneous extension of the knee. One solution is to wrap the leg in the AFO with a fabric gaiter which maintains knee extension. An alternative is to make low temperature plastic KAFOs for the legs. These are often applied in conjunction with other treatments aiming to increase the range of knee extension; the orthosis for each leg can also be connected with an abduction bar to control hip rotation.

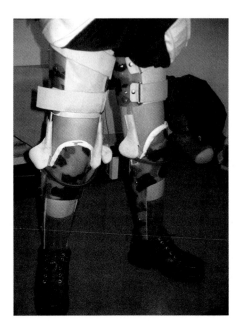

Fig. 6.19 Non-adjustable knee support riveted to side of AFO, foot and ankle are threaded through the gap between knee and AFO sections to put on and take off the KAFO.

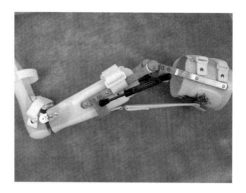

Fig. 6.20 KAFOs capable of generating active corrective forces can be used as part of a therapeutic regimen to increase range of knee joint motion.

KAFO designs to prevent or correct deformity may incorporate an incremental locking hinge, such as a dial-lock, that can be fixed in a series of increasingly extended positions. This type of orthosis can accommodate changes in the range of movement in the child's leg over time. Recently developed orthotic hinges that are capable of generating active forces may be more effective for correcting limb deformities than static orthoses. The active forces generated using compressed gas pistons or coiled springs may be more effective at a physiological level for increasing muscle length (Fig. 6.20).

Hip–knee–ankle–foot orthoses (HKAFOs)

HKAFOs TO IMPROVE FUNCTION

To enable standing hip and knee extension can be maintained using a force applied posterior to the pelvis at the sacrum which is simultaneously resisted by other forces applied anteriorly at the knees and chest and posterior to the heels (Fig. 6.21). This design constitutes the HKAFO and is useful once a child has head control and wants to achieve upright standing. The HKAFO can be attached to a heavy and broad support base to provide the stability required for a standing frame. An early version of these orthoses was the Parapodium (Motloch 1971); however, a variety of modular and custom-made standing-frame designs are now available. Simple standing-frames offer children with profound weakness the opportunity to experience upright weight-bearing posture at an age-appropriate time. It is possible to accommodate fixed hip and knee contractures of up to 30°, but in these situations heel raises should be included so that the feet are supported. Leg-length discrepancy must be accommodated to prevent pelvic obliquity. Provision of a table at the correct height can also make standing an enjoyable and stimulating activity as well as providing physiological benefits (Fig. 6.22). Upright locomotion is a worthwhile goal for children who achieve standing, as it is an activity that offers a different perception of the environment, greater independence and is also a useful form of exercise. Once stabilization of the hip joint has been accomplished, with similar force systems as in standing, then upright locomotion is possible providing the child has some control of their head, arms and trunk. This will usually be achieved using a swing-through gait, swivel-walking or assisted reciprocal ambulation. The Parapodium design has evolved to include hip and knee joints that can be unlocked

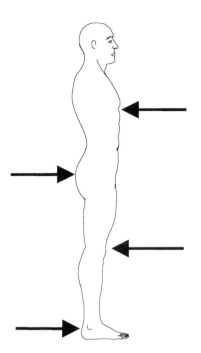

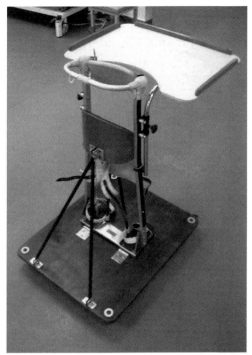

Fig. 6.21 A combination of *three-point pressure* force systems can be used to prevent hip and knee flexion and maintain an upright posture in HKAFOs.

Fig. 6.22 Standing-frame with tray attachment.

simultaneously; these are known as the Rochester or Toronto Mark II Parapodiums (see Fig. 11.2). The base plate of the Parapodium can be modified to include a mechanism to permit swivel-walking.

Swivel-walkers
Swivel-walkers consist of a standing-frame (ORLAU or Salford type) fixed to a broad heavy-base plate (Stallard et al. 1978) (Fig. 6.23). The weight of the base plate lowers the height of the centre of gravity and the frame supporting the body maintains the position of the centre of mass over the base of support. Underneath the base are two footplates mounted on bearings and offset so that either only one can be flat on the floor at any time whilst large enough to still provide extrinsic stability in this position. Providing the centre of gravity is forward of the bearing centre, when the child leans or rotates their head, arms and trunk so that only one footplate is on the supporting surface, the base plate will rotate forward on the unsupported side. Using this method only minimal coordination is required to facilitate locomotion and no walking aid is required.

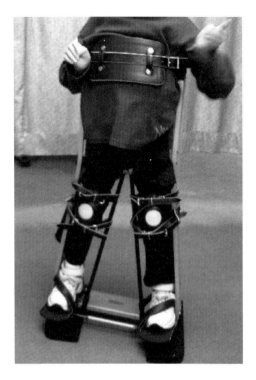

Fig. 6.23 Swivel-walker.

RECIPROCAL WALKING ORTHOSES

Swing-through and reciprocal gait require adequate upper-limb and trunk strength, especially of the latissimus dorsi muscles, and coordination to use crutches or other walking aids. Swing through gait is facilitated by HKAFOs that stabilize the whole lower body as one segment so that the upper strength can be utilized to lift the body and orthosis off the floor to swing forward. The considerable energy expenditure involved in swing-through gait renders it impossible for many children, especially when encumbered with even lightweight orthoses. The most energy-efficient and appropriate orthosis for children with inadequate hip control will usually be one of the designs of reciprocating gait orthoses. In essence, reciprocal gait requires the hip of stance limb to be extending while the hip of swing limb is flexing. This means the orthosis predominately suitable for children with flaccid limbs as spasticity impedes the efficiency of hip flexion and extension.

Scrutton (1971) and his colleagues (1967) were the first to develop polyplanar orthotic hip hinges and to connect the left and right hinges using dual cables. From these designs the first commercial reciprocating gait orthosis (RGO) system achieved reciprocal ambulation by linking the moulded plastic leg sections with two cables that flexed one hip hinge when the other extended and vice versa (Douglas et al. 1983). More recent versions of the RGO achieve adequate propulsion using either a stiffer single cable (advanced RGO) (Lissens et al. 1993) (Fig. 6.24) or rigid bars (isocentric RGO) (Campbell 1990) (Fig. 6.25) to coordinate the movement of both orthotic hip hinges. In all types of interconnected

61

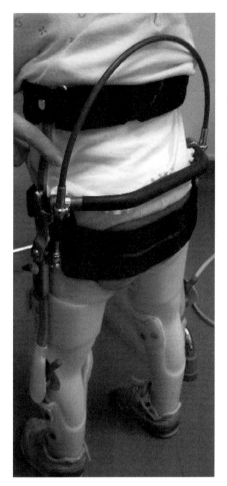
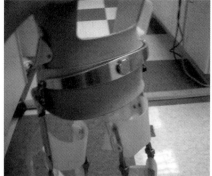
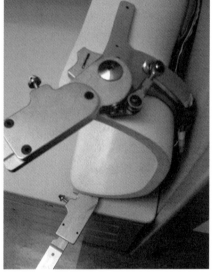

Fig. 6.24 Junior advanced reciprocating gait orthosis (ARGO).

Fig. 6.25 Isocentric RGO.

reciprocating gait orthoses, the power to flex the swinging leg comes from the ground reaction of the walking aid causing extension of the standing hip and hence flexion of the opposite hip to advance the body.

In the UK, at the Orthotic Research and Locomotion Assessment Unit (ORLAU), the hip-guidance orthosis (HGO), later commercially renamed the Parawalker, was developed to overcome the same activity limitation using a different orthotic solution (Rose et al. 1981) (Fig. 6.26). The HGO does not use cables and does not directly interconnect the motions of the orthotic hip hinges. Instead, the unloaded limb of the HGO swings forward due to the extra weight afforded by heavy footplates together with hip extension of the stance limb powered by the reaction of the ground through the walking aid and upper limbs (Butler et al. 1984, Major et al. 2001). The hip hinges themselves are rigidly connected and

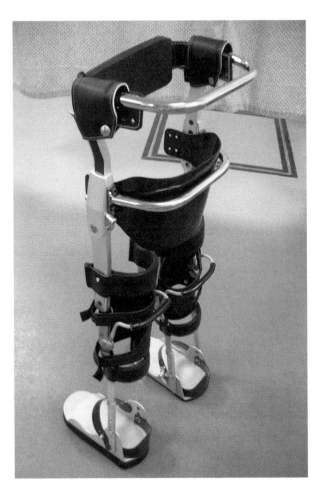

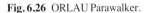**Fig. 6.26** ORLAU Parawalker.

adduction of the stance and swinging limb due to bending is resisted by the rigidity of the sidebars. As the HGO is worn over clothes it is relatively easy for children to move into position and fasten it themselves.

CONVENTIONAL HKAFOS
This chapter has so far predominately considered contemporary plastic orthoses rather than the conventional metal and leather orthoses they replaced. Plastic orthoses are favoured largely because they are light, easy to fabricate and inexpensive. However there will be occasional circumstances when conventional designs may be preferred. In the case of HKAFOs, this may be when the modular orthoses such as the swivel-walker or reciprocal walking devices are not available. The biomechanical principles to enable standing are the same, requiring forces to be applied to the anterior chest, posterior pelvis, anterior knee and posterior heel; the hip hinge must be sufficiently stiff to resist adduction. Orthotic hip hinges may lock in extension for standing and be unlocked for sitting; in addition some hinges can

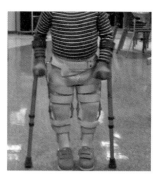

Fig. 6.27 Conventional HKAFO.

be unlocked to also permit abduction which can be an advantage when a catheter is used for urinary drainage. The sacral band must be shaped sufficiently low around the buttocks to ensure that the child's bottom cannot evade the force required to maintain hip extension. Conventional HKAFOs (Fig. 6.27) require advanced metal and leatherworking skills and are extremely time-consuming to manufacture. All metal sections must be shaped by hand to produce the substructure and then padded and covered with leather which is often hand-stitched. The additional cost of purchasing a modular design may therefore be offset by the reduced labour required to build a conventional orthosis as well as providing greater ease of use and efficiency for walking.

HKAFOs to Prevent or Correct Deformity
Total body control may be required in infancy or when significant disability is present. A low-temperature total body splint is used to control hip, knee and ankle posture in young children with myelomeningocoele after surgery or at night. Sleeping systems that control or accommodate gross deformity are also becoming part of 24-hour postural management programmes for children with cerebral palsy.

Hip orthoses (HpOs)

HpOs to Improve Function
So far in the lower limb, the orthoses described had adequate length of lever and acted in a single plane, for instance either side of the knee joint. However, as explained elsewhere in more detail (Morris 2003), the hip joint moves in all three planes and frequently one hip joint cannot be considered separately from the lower spine and the opposite hip. To make orthotic design more difficult the pelvis is irregular in shape and provides only short leverage.

Abducting the hips can be used to increase the size of the base of support and improve stability in sitting. The 'standing, walking and sitting hip-abduction' (SWASH) orthosis (Fig. 6.28) comprises a pelvic section with a posteriorly mounted curved connecting bar joined to thigh cuffs. The SWASH allows wider hip abduction when the hip is flexed, hence helping sitting stability, but a slightly less abducted position when the hip is extended. Although the SWASH may be useful to hold the knees apart during activities such as crawling and walking, the orthosis has only a circumferential containment of the pelvis. The

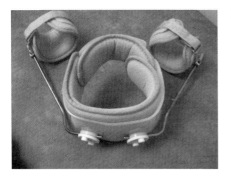

Fig. 6.28 SWASH orthosis.

limited efficacy of the SWASH to control pelvic tilt, rotation and obliquity must hinder its true control of hip abduction.

HpOs to Prevent or Correct Deformity

To maintain the hip joint in its position of maximum containment, the hip is flexed and abducted. This is a treatment modality used for neonates and infants with hip instability. HpOs such as the commonly used Pavlik harness use the superior aspect of the trunk to provide a counterforce to flexing and abducting forces applied at the thigh cuff. These orthoses are discussed in more detail in *Chapter 7*, which describes the orthotic management of congenital deformities. Maintaining hip abduction with older children is more difficult and creates psychosocial issues. The Scottish Rite hip orthosis was developed for this purpose; the combination of telescopic connecting bar and rotary motion at the thigh cuffs permits a child to walk reciprocally with both hips held abducted. However, the clinical benefits of using this orthosis must be sufficiently great to warrant imposing such an unnatural posture on a child that may otherwise walk with a regular, if antalgic, gait.

Following hip-reconstruction surgery the hip may need to be positioned in 30° of unilateral hip abduction (combined 60° angle) and 30° of hip flexion. Traditionally this would be achieved using a plaster hip spica cast. The use of an orthosis in these instances may overcome some of the complications associated with using hip spica casts, such as hygiene, pressure sores and changing wound-dressings. An alternative to the hip spica is to use a custom-moulded, one-piece plastic 'trough' that with Velcro straps encases the posterior trunk, pelvis and thighs to just proximal to the knees or ankle. This HpO can be fabricated on the child immediately after surgery using one of the lightweight plastics that can moulded at low temperatures. One disadvantage of this design is that the hip posture is not easily adjusted once the orthosis is made. The most versatile design includes a pelvic section connected rigidly to the thigh cuffs using an orthotic hinge that allows incremental adjustment (Fig. 6.29); this hip hinge can be locked in variable fixed positions in both the sagittal and coronal planes.

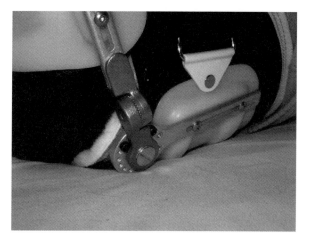

Fig. 6.29 Maple-leaf orthosis allows incremental adjustment and locking of hip flexion, extension and abduction.

References

Anthony RJ (1991) *The Manufacture and Use of the Functional Foot Orthosis*. New York: Karger.

Butler PB Major RE Patrick JH (1984) The technique of reciprocal walking using the hip guidance orthosis (HGO) with crutches. *Prosthet Orthot Int* **8**: 33–8.

Campbell JW, Inman VT (1974) Treatment of plantar fasciitis and calcaneal spurs with the UCBL shoe insert. *Clin Orthop* **103**: 57–62.

Campbell JH (1990) Reciprocating gait orthosis with linear bearing. *J Assoc Child Orthot Clin* **25**: 2–5.

Douglas R, Larson PF, D'Ambrosia R, McCall RE (1983) The LSU reciprocation-gait orthosis. *Orthopedics* **6**: 834–9.

Lissens MA, Peeraer L, Tirez B, Lysens R (1993) Advanced reciprocating gait orthosis (ARGO) in paraplegic patients. *Eur J Phys Med Rehab* **3**: 147.

Major RE Stallard J Rose GK (1981) The dynamics of walking using the Hip Guidance Orthosis (HGO) with crutches. *Prosth Orthot Int* **5**: 19–22.

Meadows CB (1984) *The influence of polypropylene ankle–foot orthoses on the gait of cerebral palsied children*. PhD thesis, University of Strathclyde.

Morris C (2003) Orthotic management of hip pathologies. In: Scrutton D, Banta J, editors. *Hip Disorders in Childhood*. London: Mac Keith Press.

Motloch W (1971) The parapodium: an orthotic device for neuromuscular disorders. *Artif Limbs* **15**: 36–47.

Philps JW (1995) *The Functional Foot Orthosis*. Edinburgh: Churchill Livingstone.

Root ML, Orien WP, Weed JH, Huighes RJ (1971) *Biomechanical Evaluation of the Foot*. Los Angeles: Clinical Biomechanics Corporation.

Rose, GK Stallard J Sankarankutty M (1981) Clinical evaluation of spina bifida patients using hip guidance orthosis. *Dev Med Child Neurol* **23**: 30–40.

Scrutton DR, Robson P, Davies RM (1967) Polyplanar hip joint for use in lower limb bracing. *Nature* **213**: 950–2.

Scrutton D (1971) A reciprocating brace with polyplanar hip hinges used on spina bifida children. *Physiotherapy* **57**: 61–6.

Stallard J, Rose GK, Farmer IR (1978) The ORLAU swivel walker. *Prosthet Orthot Int* **2**: 35–42.

7
CONGENITAL DEFORMITIES

Christopher Morris and Luciano Dias

Congenital deformities include any developmental malformations of the body structure that are diagnosed at birth or prior to birth through prenatal screening. These anomalies range from relatively minor local musculoskeletal impairments to significant orthopaedic problems as well as disorders of other systems. This chapter addresses how orthoses can play a part in the physical management of some isolated deformities and also several syndromes which manifest with physical problems.

Metatarsus adductus
This is generally an isolated positional deformity where the forefoot is adducted relative to the hindfoot at the tarso–metatarsal joints and often resolves without treatment in the first few months of life (Bleck 1982). The presence of a transverse plantar crease indicates a more severe deformity. The prognosis depends upon the severity and flexibility of the deformity and therefore it is these factors that influence treatment. If the deformity is mild, then initial treatment should be involve stretching exercises to abduct the forefoot; the regimen should be undertaken by the parents 30–40 times, three or four times every day. If the deformity has not resolved when the infant is 2 months old then serial casting is used to correct the adduction. The short leg cast is changed every 1–2 weeks until full correction is achieved (usually after 4–6 weeks). The corrected position may then be maintained either in ordinary boots or high topped shoes, special 'reverse-last' footwear (where the forefoot is more abducted than usual), or ankle-foot orthoses (AFOs) moulded to hold the forefoot in maximal abduction.

Talipes equinovarus
Congenital talipes equinovarus (CTEV), or clubfoot, involves elements of hindfoot equinus and varus, midfoot cavus and forefoot adduction (Fig. 7.1). The condition is frequently an isolated pathology but can be associated with other conditions or chromosome abnormalities. CTEV is frequently seen in infants with myelomenigocoele or arthrogryposis. The distinction may be made between a postural deformity which is flexible and more severe rigid structural deformity. Several classification systems have been proposed for grading the severity of CTEV such as the Dimeglio system (Dimeglio et al. 1995), which has been found to the most reliable of the systems available (Wainwright et al. 2002).

A precise serial-casting technique undertaken by the orthopaedic surgeon following the Ponseti method (Ponseti and Campos, 1972) is usually the first line of intervention for all types of CTEV. The method involves applying a plaster cast above the knee to maintain

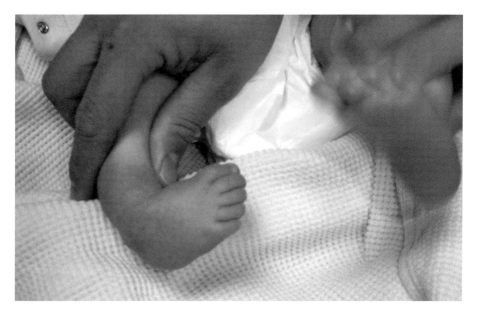

Fig. 7.1 Talipes equinovarus deformity.

the knee flexed to 90°, then first correcting the cavus element of the deformity by supination of the forefoot and at the same time abducting the forefoot and correcting the hindfoot varus (Ponsetti 1996). Correction of equinus is left till last and is done by percutaneous Achilles tendon tenotomy. Prevention of recurrence is then achieved using boots attached to a bar (similar to those first described by Denis Browne) which externally rotate the foot to about 60° and used until the children is 4 years old to maintain the ankle and foot in a corrected position at night (Fig. 7.2).

Some children with rigid CTEV or those with neuromuscular aetiology do not respond to conservative management and require more extensive surgery that may include posterior release or posterior–medial–lateral release. This is usually considered when the infant is 6–10 months old. A cast is applied immediately after surgery; following removal of that cast an AFO is used at night to maintain the foot correction, although some children such as those with arthrogryposis and myelomeningocoele also need the AFO during the day. Some suggestions for design of AFOs for children with CTEV were provided by Athearn and colleagues (1995).

There is a fine line between undercorrection and overcorrection of the deformity. When undercorrection occurs and the deformity persists but is flexible, then a supportive boot with a lateral flare to the heel will discourage inversion and adduction (Fig. 7.3); if overcorrection results in a planovalgus deformity, then the foot posture can be controlled using a polypropylene foot orthosis (Fig. 7.4). Longer-term orthotic management of CTEV may also include, in unilateral cases, provision of a toe filler insole to compensate for the smaller foot to enable shoes of the same size to be worn.

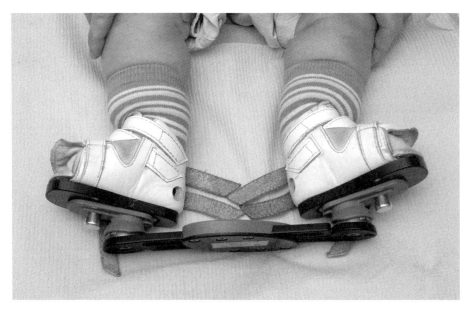

Fig. 7.2 Denis Browne 'boots-on-bar' type of orthosis used to externally rotate the foot following surgery for CTEV.

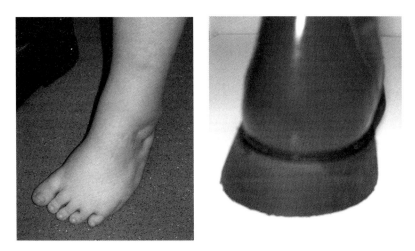

Fig. 7.3 Residual flexible deformity after surgery for CTEV can be controlled with supportive footwear and a lateral flare to the heel.

Fig. 7.4
Overcorrection can result in a planovalgus foot deformity which can be controlled using a foot orthosis.

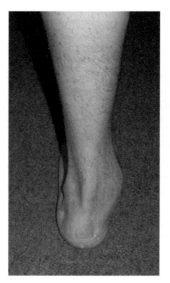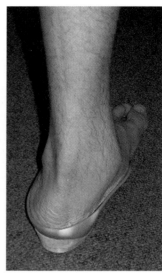

Vertical talus

Congenital vertical talus is a rare type of foot deformity. The hindfoot is in equinus, the talus is in a vertical position and the navicular is subluxed dorsally in relation to the talus. Treatment with casting or foot orthoses may improve foot alignment but conservative treatment frequently fails and surgical treatment is indicated around the age of 6–10 months. Following surgery a solid AFO is used to provide optimal correction with the foot in a functional position.

Talipes calcaneovalgus

Calcaneovalgus deformity (Fig. 7.5) principally involves excessive dorsiflexion of the ankle and is associated with abduction of the forefoot and is frequently a postural deformity. The deformity usually responds to manipulation however occasionally serial casting, splinting with low-temperature plastics or an AFO may be used as an adjunct to physical therapy.

Tibial pseudarthrosis

Pseudarthrosis of the tibia leads to anterior bowing and fractures and is associated with neurofibromatosis. The standard posterior shell of an AFO can be augmented with an anterior shell to protect the tibia and in a limited effort to limit the anterior bowing. Surgery may be required to achieve union and correct alignment however there may be a need to protect the tibia until the end of growth (Fig. 7.6).

Developmental dysplasia of the hip

The term developmental dysplasia of the hip (DDH) is preferred to congenital dislocation because (1) the impairment is not always detectable at birth, and (2) includes a spectrum of joint instability ranging from subluxation to dislocation. Most children are screened soon

70

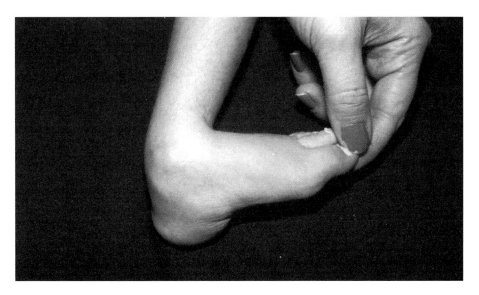

Fig. 7.5 Calcaneovalgus deformity.

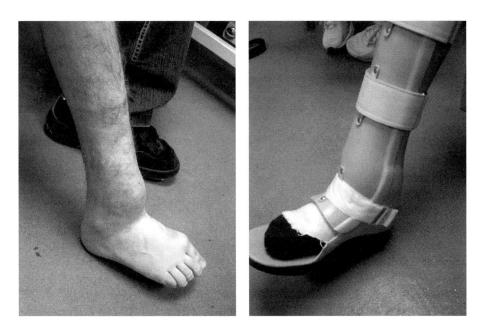

Fig. 7.6 A bivalved AFO used to protect tibial pseudarthrosis.

after birth for signs of hip dislocation using either Barlow's test or Ortalani's manoeuvre. Infants at risk should then be screened using hip ultrasound as this tends to reduce intervention without any adverse effect on outcomes or complications (Elbourne et al. 2002). Children with hip instability in the first 6 months of life are typically treated using the Pavlik harness to maintain the hip in a flexed position of 100° and abduction and limited adduction while still allowing the infant to kick their legs (Ramsey et al. 1976) (Fig. 7.7a). Application of the harness is usually undertaken by the orthopaedic surgeon rather than the orthotist or physiotherapist.

Ongoing monitoring of the hip using ultrasound while the child is using the harness is recommended beginning with an ultrasound after 1 week (Taylor and Clarke 1997). If reduction is not achieved after 3 weeks then another type of treatment should be used. This is because use of the harness can then cause significant posterior displacement of the hip, leading to increased dysplasia of the posterior acetabulum and making reduction even more difficult. The end point of using the Pavlik harness is reached using an ultrasound in which the Alpha angle should be around 60°; in the newborn period the average time in the harness is about 6 weeks. Other types of hip orthoses include the von Rosen design (Hadlow 1979) and Frejka pillow (Lempicki et al. 1990); the Denis Browne hip orthosis (Browne 1948) (Fig. 7.7b) is often appropriate for older children.

Arthrogryposis multiplex congenita
Children with arthrogryposis multiplex congenita are born with multiple joint deformities associated with muscle and joint contractures (Fig. 7.8). The syndrome describes the phenotype and therefore includes a range of conditions with different aetiology (Jones 1997). Early treatment aims to increase the range of motion available at joints although surgery is often necessary to correct deformities such as talipes equinovarus, knee contractures and hip dislocation. After surgical correction of talipes equinovarus, an AFO should be used day and night. If standing is to be a realistic objective then the knees and hips need to be

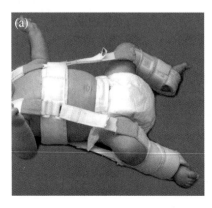 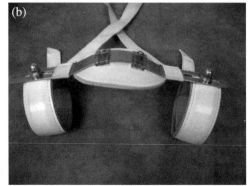

Fig. 7.7 Hip orthoses used to for developmental dysplasia of the hip: (a) Pavlik harness, and (b) Denis Browne hip orthosis.

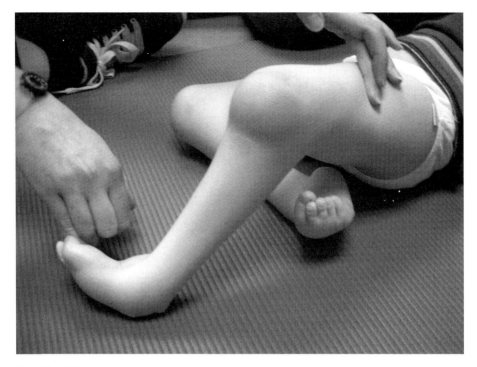

Fig. 7.8 Stiff hip- and knee-flexion deformities and talipes equinovarus are characteristics of children with arthrogryposis multiplex congenita; these deformities are usually corrected by surgery to enable orthoses to be fitted.

maintained in as extended position as possible (Robinson et al. 1984). Some children with arthrogryposis may require the help of a standing-frame, knee–ankle–foot orthosis (KAFO) or hip–knee–ankle–foot orthosis (HKAFO) to enable standing and walking (Fig. 7.9); for these children the orthosis will be lighter and less bulky if the orthotic knee hinge is not included, as the hinge serves no purpose unless there is some reasonable range of flexion available.

Osteogenesis imperfecta
Osteogenesis imperfecta is syndrome resulting from a genetic defect that impairs the body's ability to produce collagen, rendering bones that are vulnerable to break easily. The absence or poor quality of collagen fibres also manifests as joint laxity and hyperextensibility. There are different types of the condition that include a broad range of severity from just one or two fractures to, at worst, death in infancy. Treatment primarily includes pharmacological interventions that aim to increase bone density and strength. Orthotic intervention using AFOs and KAFOs can be helpful to maintain structural alignment and protect the limbs during standing and walking (Fig. 7.10).

73

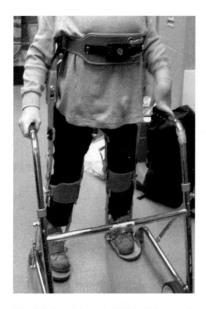 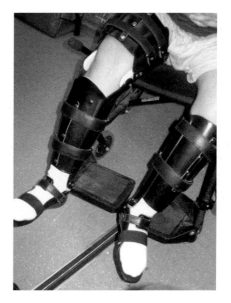

Fig. 7.9 Provision of a HKAFO Parawalker enables a child with arthrogryposis multiplex congenital to stand and walk.

Fig. 7.10 A child with Osteogenesis Imperfecta using a KAFO and AFO for protection and to maintain structural alignment during standing; hinges at the ankle and knee allow free motion in the sagittal plane.

Down syndrome

Children with Down syndrome carry an extra copy of chromosome 21 (Jones 1997). The risk of the condition is associated with older maternal age at birth, but children with Down syndrome are born to mothers of all ages. The children often have delayed gross-motor development. The musculoskeletal problems arise due to joint laxity and hypotonia and these are often compounded by excessive weight gain and obesity. There is a need to ensure that children are as active as possible to avoid excessive weight gain. Foot orthoses such as heel cups often help to improve the alignment and functioning of the foot and ankle during standing and walking.

Marfan syndrome

Children with Marfan syndrome characteristically have long narrow hyperextensible fingers and limbs, generalized joint laxity and a tall stature (Jones 1997). The joint laxity frequently results in flexible but nonetheless profound planovalgus foot deformities and the unusual length and narrow width of the foot can create problems finding suitably fitting footwear (Fig. 7.11). Children with Marfan syndrome therefore often benefit from ethylene vinyl acetate (EVA) or polypropylene foot orthoses to improve the foot and ankle posture and these orthoses also help to take up space in the footwear. Sometimes help is required to find shoes that fit. As well as foot problems a number of children with Marfan syndrome develop kyphosis and scoliosis. This may be treated with a thoracolumbar sacral orthosis (TLSO)

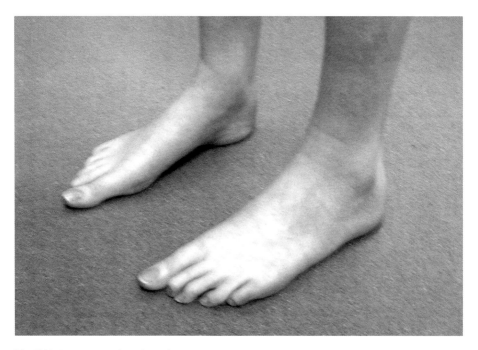

Fig. 7.11 Long narrow feet often with substantial planovalgus deformity are characteristically associated with Marfan syndrome.

to limit progression of deformity as the child grows but any significant scoliosis will usually require a spinal fusion. Those affected by Marfan syndrome are also susceptible to ocular and cardiac problems.

Other syndromes

A number of syndromes cause children physical problems which often benefit from orthotic intervention such as Lowe, Williams, Stickler and Angelman syndromes. Principally the musculoskeletal problems are joint laxity and hypo-extensibility combined with muscle hypotonia and weakness. These problems are usually most noticeable around the foot and ankle and cause or exacerbate difficulties in standing balance and walking. The provision of AFOs or FOs in these instances often improves children's stability and functioning as their abilities develop.

References

Athearn JN, Case JS, Roberts JM (1995) Impression techniques and model modification of a custom-molded ankle–foot orthosis for the idiopathic clubfoot. *J Prosthet Orthot* **7**: 91–5.

Bleck EE (1982) Developmental orthopaedics. III: Toddlers. *Dev Med Child Neurol* **24**: 533–5.

Browne D (1948) The treatment of congenital dislocation of the hip. *Proc Royal Soc Med* **41**: 388–90.

Dimeglio A, Bensahel H, Souchet P, Mazeau P, Bonnet F (1995) Classification of clubfoot. *J Pediatr Orthop B* **7**: 129–36.

Elbourne D, Dezateux C, Arthur R, Clarke NM, Gray A, King A, Quinn A, Gardner F, Russell G, UK Collaborative Hip Trial Group (2002) Ultrasonography in the diagnosis and management of developmental hip dysplasia (UK Hip Trial): clinical and economic results of a multicentre randomised controlled trial. *Lancet* **360**: 2009–17.

Hadlow VD (1979) Congenital dislocation of the hip over a ten-year period. *N Z Med J*: 126–8.

Jones KL (1997) *Smith's Recognizable Patterns of Human Malformation*. Philadelphia: W.B. Saunders.

Lempicki A, Wierusz-Kozlowska M, Kruczynski J (1990) Abduction treatment in late diagnosed congenital dislocation of the hip. Follow-up of 1,010 hips treated with the Frejka pillow 1967–76. *Acta Orthop Scand* Suppl. **236**: 1–30.

Ponseti IV, Campos J (1972) Observations on pathogenesis and treatment of congenital clubfoot. *Clinical Orthopaedics* **84**: 50–60.

Ponseti IV (1996) *Congenital Clubfoot. Fundamentals for Treatment*. Oxford: Oxford University Press.

Ramsey PL, Lasser S, MacEwen GD (1976) Congenital dislocation of the hip. Use of the Pavlik harness in the child during the first six months of life. *J Bone Joint Surg Am* **58**: 1000–4

Robinson RO, Cartwight R, Fixsen JA, Rockey J (1984) Arthrogryposis multiplex congenita. In: McCarthy GT, editor. *The Physically Handicapped Child*. London: Faber & Faber.

Taylor GR, Clarke NM (1997) Monitoring the treatment of developmental dysplasia of the hip with the Pavlik harness. The role of ultrasound. *J Bone Joint Surg Br* **79**: 719–23.

Wainwright AM, Auld T, Benson MK, Theologis TN (2002) The classification of congenital talipes equinovarus. *J Bone Joint Surg Br* **84**: 1020–4.

8
CONDITIONS ARISING IN CHILDHOOD

Christopher Morris and Luciano Dias

While the previous section covered congenital deformities, there are a group of deformities that arise during childhood. These problems may become symptomatic in association with some other factor, such as participating in a new activity or exercising excessively, or the anomaly may only become apparent following clinical investigation. The lower limbs are perhaps more susceptible to these types of conditions because of higher external forces acting on the body during regular activities. As such they constitute a group of 'acute' conditions that may benefit from a period of treatment with orthoses. However, other conditions arising in childhood, such as juvenile idiopathic arthritis, have a more profound prognosis and can be quite debilitating and require long-term use of orthoses.

Pes planovalgus

Planovalgus foot posture (Fig. 8.1), frequently referred to as flat foot, is a common cause of concern for parents but does not usually require treatment unless there is pain or excessive shoe wear. Observational research suggests that flat foot is in fact normal in infants, common in children and within the normal distribution of foot shapes in adults (Staheli et al. 1987). There is a higher incidence of flat feet between 2 and 4 years of age, and there is a progression of medial arch development up to the age of 8 years (Volpon 1994). In terms of orthotic management, important distinctions are made between (1) asymptomatic flexible planovalgus, (2) flexible planovalgus with symptoms, and (3) rigid planovalgus deformity.

ASYMPTOMATIC PES PLANOVALGUS

The appearance of a flexible or physiological pes planovalgus is of a normal foot when non-weight-bearing, but the midfoot pronates excessively during standing and walking and the heel may also tilt slightly into valgus. Children with flexible planovalgus often have excessive range of movement due to generalized benign joint hypermobility; examination to determine if the child has passive hyperextension of other joints, such as the knee and thumb for example, can reveal this generalized joint laxity. There is little influence from using foot orthoses on the development of foot shape during growth. A clinical trial that randomly allocated children with flexible flat feet to either a control group or one of three groups treated with special footwear, stock heel cups or custom made foot orthoses found no difference in treatment outcomes (Wenger et al. 1989). Although the number in each arm of the trial was small, the children were followed up for 3 years and all groups demonstrated an improvement in foot shape. Therefore if the foot and ankle are flexible and asymptomatic then no treatment is required, and any intervention may do more harm than good (Driano

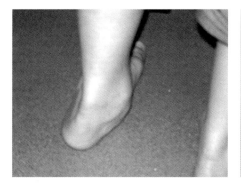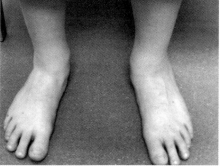

Fig. 8.1 Planovalgus foot posture is a combination of hindfoot eversion and midfoot pronation, there may also be forefoot abduction.

et al. 1998). Rather, the family should be reassured that there is no pathology. An inexpensive pair of stock insoles may be provided for a short period when parental concern is not fully allayed.

It is important to identify children presenting with planovalgus who do not have a complete range of dorsiflexion at the ankle. Although the foot and ankle may be flexible when the knee is flexed, if there is any restriction in range of dorsiflexion when the knee is extended then, during standing, the heel tends to tilt into valgus causing the midfoot to pronate excessively. Planovalgus deformity is then secondary to the reduced length of the gastrocnemius. For these children an intensive stretching regimen may be sufficient to restore range of motion at the ankle, or serial casting or a night ankle–foot orthosis (AFO) may be indicated; occasionally surgery involving gastrocnemius recession is necessary.

SYMPTOMATIC PES PLANOVALGUS
The provision of orthoses can be beneficial when symptoms of pain or excessive shoe wear occur that are associated with the planovalgus foot. Pain can result from the extra tensile stresses along the soft tissues of the medial arch or due to impingement of the lateral bony structures of the ankle or sinus tarsi area. Foot posture should first be examined non-weight-bearing and then also in standing and walking. The range of ankle motion and muscle power should be tested with the knee flexed and extended, and particularly the functioning of the tibialis posterior muscle. As described above, any restriction of dorsiflexion will exacerbate the planovalgus and should therefore be treated with stretching, night-splinting using an AFO, serial casting or surgery. Polypropylene foot orthoses can be made to a cast of the child's foot in the optimally corrected position. Increasing the depth of heel cupping within the orthosis provides greater control of the subtalar and midtarsal joints (Fig. 8.2). EVA foam foot orthoses may be more appropriate for children with moderate symptoms or tenderness (Fig. 8.3). Treatment should be reviewed after 6–12 months.

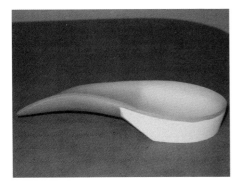 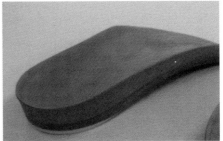

Fig. 8.2 Polypropylene foot orthosis and heel cup. **Fig. 8.3** EVA foot orthosis.

RIGID PLANOVALGUS

A rigid flat foot requires radiological evaluation to identify the cause of the reduced hind- and midfoot joint motions. Tarsal coalitions occur when the bones of the mid- and hindfoot fail to separate completely during growth and usually becomes symptomatic over the age of 10 years (Fig. 8.4). The two most common are the calcaneonavicular and mid-facet talocalcaneal bar; initial treatment with foot orthoses may help to decrease the pain, but frequently surgical excision of the coalition is required.

When the foot is not flexible then the options for orthotic intervention are limited to accommodating the best position to allow the foot to function as normally as possible. Assessment should establish the cross-planar relationships between the forefoot, hindfoot and lower leg segments. To achieve stability in stance the hindfoot must lie directly under the lower leg, however, when this is manipulated in rigid flat feet the medial forefoot often remains in a supinated position. This can be accommodated using a foot orthosis to maintain the elevation of the medial forefoot inside the shoe (sometimes termed *posting*) or if there is insufficient space then a wedge of material can also be added to the medial aspect of the external sole of the shoe. If the weight line of the body is passing too medially, outside the base of support offered by the shoe then stability is lost. If this remains after using insoles and sole wedging then the external base of shoe support can be widened medially.

Hallux valgus

Hallux valgus occurs relatively infrequently in children and although the deformity can be painful it is more often an aesthetic problem. The hallux is seen to deviate laterally and may also internally rotate during walking as the normal motion of the first metatarsophalangeal joint is disrupted. Hallux valgus is particularly exacerbated during late stance when the heel rises and the whole weight of the body and propulsive forces are borne on the forefoot; this is especially so when there is any restriction of the range of dorsiflexion of the hallux. Foot orthoses which support the medial arch and first metatarsal can reduce forces acting on the first metatarsophalangeal joint as the heel rises. However, whilst orthoses used during walking might help to reduce any associated pain, insoles are unlikely to prevent or correct

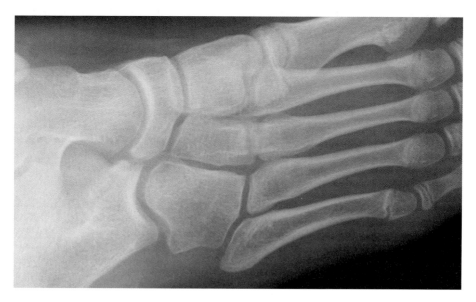

Fig. 8.4 Oblique view X-ray of the tarsal bones showing bony coalition between calcaneum and navicular.

the deformity (Kilmartin et al. 1994). There are suggestions that treatment using a plastic orthosis at night, combined with exercises, might improve the deformity (Groiso 1992); however, the evidence to support using orthoses for hallux valgus is not compelling (Ferrari 2005).

Accessory navicular

The tibialis posterior muscle attaches to the midtarsal bones around the navicular and is functionally important in maintaining the medial arch during gait. The tendon can be placed under great strain during periods of repetitive excessive pronation. In children this can lead to a traction apophysitis that presents as a tender bump over the prominent aspect of the navicular, causing pain during activities and may also rub on the shoe. The symptoms usually start after the age of 10 years. Orthotic intervention aims to reduce the strain on the apophysis by supporting the medial arch and is usually effective both in alleviating pain and allowing the additional bone to fuse. Tenderness over the affected area means the child may not tolerate a rigid plastic orthosis and a softer custom-moulded EVA insole often works well. If orthotic management is not successful then the accessory navicular should be surgically excised (Bennett et al. 1990).

Sever's disease

Sever's disease is a similar traction apophysitis affecting the heel where the Achilles tendon attaches to the calcaneum and is often associated with children who are more active in sports. Particularly vigorous activities should be avoided especially when symptoms are severe. Providing a 10–15mm silicon or polyurethane cushion is usually effective in reducing the strain on the tendon and dissipating ground reaction forces around the heel. If the condition is associated with excessive midfoot pronation then the heel cushion can be incorporated into a medial arch supporting insole. Sever's disease usually subsides over time and regular activities can be restored and the child can be weaned from the orthosis. Any lost range of dorsiflexion movement during the painful period should be recovered through a programme of stretching of the gastrocnemius and soleus muscles.

Toe-walking

Toe-walking in children has a wide range of causes and treatment varies according to the aetiology. Children with neurological problems such as cerebral palsy walk on their toes because of hypertonicity of the calf muscles. In contrast children with proximal muscle weakness, for example in the early stages of Duchenne muscular dystrophy, walk on their toes as a compensatory strategy to reduce the demands on the quadriceps. However, when toe-walking occurs without any underlying neuromuscular pathology this is termed idiopathic or habitual toe-walking (Sala et al. 1999). In some children the gait problem may be associated with speech pathology or learning disability, and these associated symptoms may be indicative of developmental delay or autism (Shulman et al. 1997).

Clinical assessment should determine whether or not the child has an equinus deformity. When at least 10° of dorsiflexion exists, then treatment with a hinged AFO preventing plantarflexion is appropriate together with gait reeducation from a therapist. When a fixed equinus contracture exists then this can usually be resolved by a serial casting programme over several weeks to increase the range of dorsiflexion. For children who have just undergone serial casting it may be more prudent to use a solid rather than hinged AFO as this will be more effective in continuing to stretch the gastrocnemius. For some children surgery is required to correct the equinus and facilitate management with AFOs. The child should be weaned from the AFOs once their gait begins to improve.

In- and out-toeing

Parents occasionally become concerned that their child is walking with his/her feet turned excessively inwards or outwards; this is called in-toeing and out-toeing. These usually fall within the broad range of normal development and require no treatment (Staheli et al. 1985). An internal foot-progression angle can be caused by greater pelvic rotation during gait, which is a natural method for increasing step length and may therefore be accentuated when the child is running. Internal foot-progression gait may also be secondary to metatarsus adductus; more frequently, however, the child may have increased femoral anteversion or internal tibial torsion affecting the foot-progression angle. The internal tibial torsion tends to resolve itself by 2 years of age, however, for children aged between 18 and 30 months it can be treated using the Denis Browne 'boots on bar' (Fig. 7.2) with the foot in 40° of external rotation (Bleck 1982), although the evidence is equivocal (Heinrich and Sharps 1991). There is no active treatment for increased femoral anteversion; the natural history is a gradual improvement right up to the age of 12–13 years and surgical treatment is rarely indicated.

Out-toeing gait in a toddler is usually caused by an external rotation 'contracture' at the hip. It gradually improves as the child continues to walk. In an older child, it can be caused by a pes planovalgus or excessive external tibial torsion. If any surgical treatment is being considered for an excessive internal or external tibial torsion, instrumented 3D gait analysis is indicated.

Tibial varum and Blount's disease

Bowleg describes the appearance of legs in which the tibia appears to be bowing laterally and is usually within the normal variation in infants; this is referred to as physiological genu varum and does not require treatment. In children over the age of 2 years with excessive genu varum one must rule out Blount's disease; this is a medial translation of the proximal tibial growth plate. A classification of severity based on X-rays was described by Langenskiold (1989). Young children aged between 2 and 4 years with the least severe forms, Langenskiold stages I and II, may respond to orthotic intervention using a knee–ankle–foot orthosis (KAFO) (Raney et al. 1998, Richards et al. 1998). The KAFO described by these authors aims to exert a lateral corrective force to the upper tibia which is countered by stabilizing the ankle in a boot, to prevent the foot being forced into valgus, and above the knee with a flange extending down over the medial condyle to protect the knee from be pushed into valgus. The orthosis is cumbersome and is intended to be worn day and night; therefore conservative treatment is challenging to the child and family. For children with stage III or higher, and those for whom orthoses are ineffective, surgical correction of alignment is achieved by proximal tibial osteotomy.

Knee pain and instability

Anterior knee pain in children is often associated with those who like sporting activities. Magnetic resonance imaging (MRI) may be required to investigate any intra-articular pathology. Knee pain may arise due to the effect of the ground reaction force acting about the knee secondary to poor foot posture or excessive pronation. There is limited evidence that the solution to anterior knee pain may be providing foot rather than knee orthoses (D'hondt et al. 2006), but this is often worth trying. A number of proprietary fabric orthoses exist that may help to provide limited external support and warmth to the knee. Lateral subluxation of the patella can cause knee pain and one treatment objective is preventing displacement of the patella using an orthosis; the difficulty is obtaining sufficient friction to stabilize the relatively small protuberance of the patella under the skin.

Legg–Calve–Perthes disease

Legg–Calve–Perthes disease, often known as Perthes, describes changes in the proximal femoral epiphysis secondary to avascular necrosis. Theoretically it makes sense to protect the hip joint of the forces and walking that could increase the deformity of the femoral head. Various orthotic solutions have been developed for Perthes, the Scottish Rite (Meehan et al. 1992), the Newington (Curtis et al. 1974), and the Toronto orthosis (Bobechko 1974). However evidence for the effectiveness of such orthoses for treating Perthes is lacking (Martinez et al. 1992) and, combined with the negative psychosocial effects (Price et al.

1988), they are now rarely used. A hip orthosis is sometimes used at night to keep the hip in abduction.

Leg-length discrepancy

A number of different orthopaedic pathologies can lead to a leg-length discrepancy (LLD). In order to maintain symmetrical posture and avoid compensatory curvature of the spine and back pain it is necessary to accommodate the LLD using some form of levelling raise or foot orthosis. A difference of up to 15 mm can be hidden inside the shoe using an internal heel elevator or insole. When the LLD exceeds this height or if the shoe is too low cut to accommodate an internal shoe raise then the additional material can be fixed to the underside of shoe. Ethylene vinyl acetate (EVA) materials enable lightweight modification of most types of shoes, often inserting the raise within the original sole of the shoe for a better appearance. The height of the heel of the shoe, or pitch, will influence the exact dimensions of the shoe raise. In order to avoid excessive pressure under the forefoot, material is added to both the sole and heel. However, because the added material will stiffen the shoe and restrict the heel from rising during gait, the raise is tapered off towards the toe end of the shoe to enable tibial advancement and the heel and toe off. When the predicted LLD exceeds 2 cm surgical treatment is indicated, either epiphysiodesis or leg lengthening.

Juvenile idiopathic arthritis

Juvenile idiopathic arthritis (JIA) is a chronic inflammatory arthropathy of unknown aetiology that begins before the child is 16 years old and persists for at least 6 weeks (Petty et al. 2004). Inflammation, swelling and stiffness of the joints, especially in the early morning, are the predominant symptoms. The principal effects of JIA on the feet are seen at the ankle, subtalar and metatarsophalangeal joints; inflammations where the muscles attach to the bones are also often problematic. Custom foot orthoses with shock absorbing properties are used to promote good ankle foot and overall posture, to improve stability and reduce pain around joints or to provide pressure relief underneath the foot (Powell et al. 2005). Elastic fabric or low-temperature plastic wrist–hand orthoses are used to stabilize the wrist and maintain optimal alignments in an effort to promote manual ability when those joints are affected. Temporary splinting is occasionally used to limit painful movement for pain relief at joints such as the elbow and knee in an effort to reduce painful symptoms and maintain range of movement (Fredriksen and Mengshoel, 2000).

Haemophilia

With active coagulation factors now widely used to treat haemophilia there is a reduced requirement for orthotic management of the secondary complications of intra-articular bleeding. Orthoses are used to immobilize affected joints and to maintain range of movement and stability in those joints. There may however still be a case for providing custom shock absorbing foot orthoses for children who have pain or instability of the ankles (Slattery and Tinley 2001).

References

Bennett GL, Weiner DS, Leighley B (1990) Surgical treatment of symptomatic accessory tarsal navicular. *J Pediatr Orthop* **10**: 445–9.

Bleck EE (1982) Developmental orthopaedics. III: Toddlers. *Dev Med Child Neurol* **24**: 533–55.

Bobechko WP (1974) The Toronto brace for Legg-Perthes disease. *Clin Orthop Relat Res* **102**: 115–17.

Curtis BH, Gunther SF, Gossling HR, Paul SW (1974) Treatment for Legg-Perthes disease with the Newington ambulation abduction brace. *J Bone Joint Surg Am* **56**: 1135–46.

D'hondt NE, Struijs PAA, Kerkhoffs GMMJ, Verheul C, Lysens R, Aufdemkampe G, Van Dijk CN (2006) Orthotic devices for treating patellofemoral pain syndrome. *Cochrane Database of Systematic Reviews* **1**.

Driano AN, Staheli L, Staheli LT (1998) Psychosocial development and corrective shoewear use in childhood. *J Pediatr Orthop* **18**: 346–9.

Ferrari J (2005) Bunions. *Clin Evid* **13**: 1377–87.

Fredriksen B, Mengshoel AM (2000) The effect of static traction and orthoses in the treatment of knee contractures in preschool children with juvenile chronic arthritis: a single-subject design. *Arthritis Care Res* **13**: 352–9.

Groiso JA (1992) Juvenile hallux valgus. A conservative approach to treatment. *J Bone Joint Surg Am* **74**: 1367–74.

Heinrich SD, Sharps CH (1991) Lower extremity torsional deformities in children: a prospective comparison of two treatment modalities. *Orthopedics* **14**: 655–9.

Kilmartin TE, Barrington RL, Wallace WA (1994) A controlled prospective trial of a foot orthosis for juvenile hallux valgus. *J Bone Joint Surg Br* **76**: 210–14.

Langenskiold A (1989) Tibia vara. A critical review. *Clin Orthop Relat Res* **246**: 195–207.

Martinez AG, Weinstein SL, Dietz FR (1992) The weight-bearing abduction brace for the treatment of Legg–Perthes disease. *J Bone Joint Surg Am* **74**: 12–21.

Meehan PL, Angel D, Nelson JM (1992) The Scottish Rite abduction orthosis for the treatment of Legg-Perthes disease. A radiographic analysis. *J Bone Joint Surg Am* **74**: 2–12.

Petty RE, Southwood TR, Manners P, Baum J, Glass DN, Goldenberg J, He X, Maldonado-Cocco J, Orozco-Alcala J, Prieur AM, Suarez-Almazor ME, Woo P, International League of Associations for Rheumatology (2004) International League of Associations for Rheumatology classification of juvenile idiopathic arthritis: second revision, Edmonton, 2001. *J Rheumatol* **31**: 390–2.

Powell M, Seid M, Szer IS (2005) Efficacy of custom foot orthotics in improving pain and functional status in children with juvenile idiopathic arthritis: a randomized trial. *J Rheumatol* **32**: 943–50.

Price CT, Day DD, Flynn JC (1998) Behavioral sequelae of bracing versus surgery for Legg–Calve–Perthes disease. *J Pediatr Orthop* **8**: 285–7.

Raney EM, Topoleski TA, Yaghoubian R, Guidera KJ, Marshall JG (1998) Orthotic treatment of infantile tibia vara. *J Pediatr Orthop* **18**: 670–4.

Richards BS, Katz DE, Sims JB (1998) Effectiveness of brace treatment in early infantile Blount's disease. *J Pediatr Orthop* **18**: 374–80.

Sala DA, Shulman LH, Kennedy RF, Grant AD, Chu ML (1999) Idiopathic toe-walking: a review. *Dev Med Child Neurol* **41**: 846–8.

Shulman LH, Sala DA, Chu ML, McCaul PR, Sandler BJ (1997) Developmental implications of idiopathic toe walking. *J Pediatr* **130**: 541–6.

Slattery M, Tinley P (2001) The efficacy of functional foot orthoses in the control of pain in ankle joint disintegration in hemophilia. *J Am Podiatr Med Assoc* **91**: 240–4.

Staheli LT, Corbett M, Wyss C, King H (1985) Lower-extremity rotational problems in children. Normal values to guide management. *J Bone Joint Surg Am* **67**: 39–47.

Staheli LT, Chew DE, Corbett M (1987) The longitudinal arch. A survey of eight hundred and eighty-two feet in normal children and adults. *J Bone Joint Surg Am* **69**: 426–8.

Volpon JB (1994) Footprint analysis during the growth period. *J Pediatr Orthop* **14**: 83–5.

Wenger DR, Mauldin D, Speck G, Morgan D, Lieber RL (1989) Corrective shoes and inserts as treatment for flexible flatfoot in infants and children. *J Bone Joint Surg Am* **71**: 800–10.

9
CEREBRAL PALSY

Christopher Morris

Cerebral palsy (CP) is the most common cause of neuromuscular physical disability in children (Surveillance of Cerebral Palsy in Europe 2000). The most recent definition is that 'cerebral palsy describes a group of permanent disorders of the development of movement and posture, causing activity limitation, that are attributed to non-progressive disturbances that occurred in the developing fetal or infant brain. The motor disorders of CP are often accompanied by disturbances of sensation, perception, cognition, communication, behaviour, by epilepsy and by secondary musculoskeletal problems' (Rosenbaum et al. 2007). The group for Surveillance of Cerebral Palsy in Europe (SCPE) have developed a coherent system for describing the primary neurological impairment, (1) by the type of motor disorder: spastic, dyskinetic, ataxic or unclassifiable; and (2) by the number of limbs affected, bilateral or hemiplegia (Surveillance of Cerebral Palsy in Europe, 2000). The terms quadriplegia for four-limb (total body) involvement and diplegia when the lower limbs are more affected than the arms, although often used, are not always easy to apply. This is especially true when the impairment is asymmetrical hence the terms asymmetrical diplegia or double hemiplegia are also used. The impact of skeletal growth during childhood can compound the primary neurological problem if muscles fail to lengthen in proportion to their adjacent long bones; and spastic muscles have been shown to grow more slowly than normal (Ziv et al. 1984). Therefore, although CP is by definition a static neurological lesion and a disorder of motor function, the phenotype has also been labelled a 'progressive neuromuscular deformity' (Graham 2002). The symptoms range from a mild gait abnormality to profound total body involvement.

A valid and reliable means of describing the severity of a child's motor impairment is provided by the Gross Motor Function Classification System (GMFCS) (Palisano et al. 1997). The GMFCS enables a child's movement abilities to be classified reliably at one of five levels, from descriptions currently provided for four age-bands: less than 2 years, 2–4 years, 4–6 years and 6–12 years; an older age-band for young people aged 13–18 years has recently been developed. Children at level I are the least affected and can achieve most the activities of their age-matched normal counterparts, perhaps with only modest qualitative differences. Conversely, children at level V are the most limited in their activities and have little ability to control their head and trunk posture to counter the effects of the motor impairment and gravity (Fig. 9.1). Although the GMFCS describes only a child's motor function, rates of functional limitation in mobility, manual dexterity, speech and vision, and to a lesser extent hearing and cognition, have been shown to correlate with GMFCS levels (Kennes et al. 2002). As children are not expected to change level over time, the

GMFCS Level I

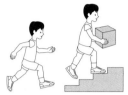

Children walk at home, school, outdoors, and in the community. Children are able to walk up and down curbs without physical assistance and stairs without the use of a railing. Children perform gross motor skills such as running and jumping but speed, balance, and coordination are limited. Children may participate in physical activities and sports depending on personal choices and environmental factors.

GMFCS Level II

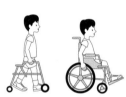

Children walk in most settings. Children may experience difficulty walking long distances and balancing on uneven terrain, inclines, in crowded areas, confined spaces or when carrying objects. Children walk up and down stairs holding onto a railing or with physical assistance if there is no railing. Outdoors and in the community, children may walk with physical assistance, a hand-held mobility device, or use wheeled mobility when travelling long distances. Children have at best only minimal ability to perform gross motor skills such as running and jumping. Limitations in performance of gross motor skills may necessitate adaptations to enable participation in physical activities and sports

GMFCS Level III

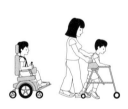

Children walk using a hand-held mobility device in most indoor settings. When seated, children may require a seat belt for pelvic alignment and balance. Sit-to-stand and floor-to-stand transfers require physical assistance of a person or support surface. When travelling long distances, children use some form of wheeled mobility. Children may walk up and down stairs holding onto a railing with supervision or physical assistance. Limitations in walking may necessitate adaptations to enable participation in physical activities and sports including self-propelling a manual wheelchair or powered mobility.

GMFCS Level IV

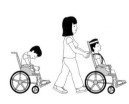

Children use methods of mobility that require physical assistance or powered mobility in most settings. Children require adaptive seating for trunk and pelvic control and physical assistance for most transfers. At home, children use floor mobility (roll, creep, or crawl), walk short distances with physical assistance, or use powered mobility. When positioned, children may use a body support walker at home or school. At school, outdoors, and in the community, children are transported in a manual wheelchair or use powered mobility. Limitations in mobility necessitate adaptations to enable participation in physical activities and sports, including physical assistance and/or powered mobility.

GMFCS Level V

Children are transported in a manual wheelchair in all settings. Children are limited in their ability to maintain antigravity head and trunk postures and control arm and leg movements. Assistive technology is used to improve head alignment, seating, standing, and and/or mobility but limitations are not fully compensated by equipment. Transfers require complete physical assistance of an adult. At home, children may move short distances on the floor or may be carried by an adult. Children may achieve self-mobility using powered mobility with extensive adaptations for seating and control access. Limitations in mobility necessitate adaptations to enable participation in physical activities and sports including physical assistance and using powered mobility.

Fig. 9.1 Descriptions of Gross Motor Function Classification System between 6 and 12 years (*above*), and from 12 to 18 years old (*opposite*) (text copyright Bob Palisano, Peter Rosenbaum, Doreen Bartlett and Can Child Centre for Disability Research; illustrations copyright Kerr Graham, Bill Reid and Adrienne Harvey).

GMFCS Level I

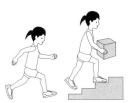

Youth walk at home, school, outdoors, and in the community. Youth are able to walk up and down curbs without physical assistance and stairs without the use of a railing. Youth perform gross motor skills such as running and jumping but speed, balance, and coordination are limited. Youth may participate in physical activities and sports depending on personal choices and environmental factors.

GMFCS Level II

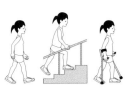

Youth walk in most settings. Environmental factors (such as uneven terrain, inclines, long distances, time demands, weather, and peer acceptability) and personal preference influence mobility choices. At school or work, youth may walk using a hand-held mobility device for safety. Outdoors and in the community, youth may use wheeled mobility when traveling long distances. Youth walk up and down stairs holding a railing or with physical assistance if there is no railing. Limitations in performance of gross motor skills may necessitate adaptations to enable participation in physical activities and sports.

GMFCS Level III

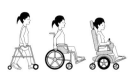

Youth are capable of walking using a hand-held mobility device. Compared to individuals in other levels, youth in Level III demonstrate more variability in methods of mobility depending on physical ability and environmental and personal factors. When seated, youth may require a harness or restraint around the waist for pelvic alignment and balance. Sit-to-stand and floor-to-stand transfers require physical assistance from a person or support surface. At school, youth may self-propel a manual wheelchair or use powered mobility. Outdoors and in the community, youth are transported in a wheelchair or use powered mobility. Youth may walk up and down stairs holding onto a railing with supervision or physical assistance. Limitations in walking may necessitate adaptations to enable participation in physical activities and sports including self-propelling a manual wheelchair or powered mobility.

GMFCS Level IV

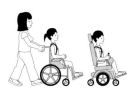

Youth use wheeled mobility in most settings. Youth require adaptive seating for pelvic and trunk control. Physical assistance from 1 or 2 persons is required for transfers. Youth may support weight with their legs to assist with standing transfers. Indoors, youth may walk short distances with physical assistance, use wheeled mobility, or, when positioned, use a body support walker. Youth are physically capable of operating a powered wheelchair. When a powered wheelchair is not feasible or available, youth are transported in a manual wheelchair. Limitations in mobility necessitate adaptations to enable participation in physical activities and sports, including physical assistance and/or powered mobility.

GMFCS Level V

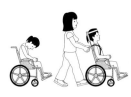

Youth are transported in a manual wheelchair in all settings. Youth are limited in their ability to maintain antigravity head and trunk postures and control arm and leg movements. Assistive technology is used to improve head alignment, seating, standing, and mobility but limitations are not fully compensated by equipment. Physical assistance from 1 or 2 persons or a mechanical lift is required for transfers. Youth may achieve self-mobility using powered mobility with extensive adaptations for seating and control access. Limitations in mobility necessitate adaptations to enable participation in physical activities and sports including physical assistance and using powered mobility.

Fig. 9.1 (*contd*) For caption, see opposite.

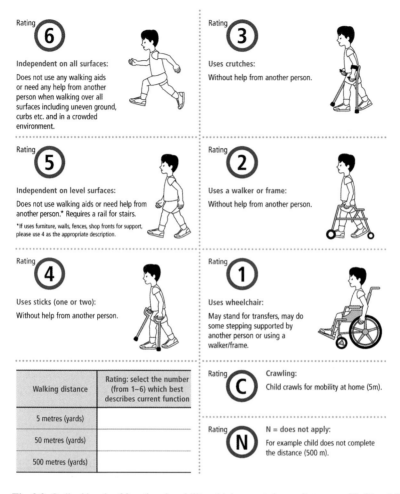

Rating 6

Independent on all surfaces:

Does not use any walking aids or need any help from another person when walking over all surfaces including uneven ground, curbs etc. and in a crowded environment.

Rating 5

Independent on level surfaces:

Does not use walking aids or need help from another person.* Requires a rail for stairs.

*If uses furniture, walls, fences, shop fronts for support, please use 4 as the appropriate description.

Rating 4

Uses sticks (one or two):

Without help from another person.

Rating 3

Uses crutches:

Without help from another person.

Rating 2

Uses a walker or frame:

Without help from another person.

Rating 1

Uses wheelchair:

May stand for transfers, may do some stepping supported by another person or using a walker/frame.

Rating C

Crawling:

Child crawls for mobility at home (5m).

Rating N

N = does not apply:

For example child does not complete the distance (500 m).

Walking distance	Rating: select the number (from 1–6) which best describes current function
5 metres (yards)	
50 metres (yards)	
500 metres (yards)	

Fig. 9.2 Ordinal levels of functional mobility which are rated over distances of 5, 50 and 500 m to create a profile of children's walking ability using the Functional Mobility Scale. (Copyright Kerr Graham, Bill Reid and Adrienne Harvey.)

GMFCS can be used as a prognostic instrument for predicting motor development for children with CP (Rosenbaum et al. 2002). The GMFCS has had a profound impact on the design of related observational and experimental research and has become the standard way for describing children with CP (Morris and Bartlett 2004).

The Functional Mobility Scale (FMS) is a recently developed method for classifying children's walking ability according to their need for assistive devices across three distances: 5, 50 and 500 metres (Graham et al. 2004) (Fig. 9.2). In contrast to the GMFCS, in which children are not expected to change levels even with intervention, the FMS is sensitive to detecting functional changes within individual children. The FMS therefore offers a valid method for measuring outcomes after interventions such as instance orthopaedic surgery.

Upper-limb function can be classified using the Manual Ability Classification System (MACS) (Eliasson et al. 2006). The MACS is similar in concept to the GMFCS where a child's ability to handle objects is classified in to one of five levels taking typical age-appropriate factors into account. The Gross Motor Function Measure (GMFM) and Pediatric Evaluation of Disability Inventory (PEDI) are instruments that have been shown to be responsive to measuring change in functioning in children with cerebral palsy (Vos-Vromans et al. 2005); the GMFM has been shown to be specifically responsive to change related to using orthoses (Russell and Gorter 2005).

Treatment goals

Orthotic intervention plays an important part in the management of children with cerebral palsy but the subject cannot easily be discussed in isolation; it is essential to recognise that orthoses are part of multimodal therapeutic programmes together with other medical, surgical and therapeutic interventions. The aims of lower-limb orthotic management of CP were identified by a consensus conference convened by the International Society of Prosthetics and Orthotics (ISPO) as (1) to correct and / or prevent deformity, (2) to provide a base of support; (3) to facilitate training in skills; and (4) to improve the efficiency of gait (Condie and Meadows 1995). A degree of compromise may be necessary in planning orthotic intervention, as orthoses prescribed to prevent or correct deformities or improve gait efficiency may restrict movements and limit other activities. The ISPO consensus conference considered orthotic intervention as relating to three levels of function: (1) the pre-standing child, recognizing that this may be the highest level of activity for some children, (2) the standing child, and (3) the walking child (Condie and Meadows 1995).

To Correct and/or Prevent Deformity

Flexible joint deformities, due to gravity or unbalanced muscle forces, can be corrected passively and the position maintained using orthoses. Fixed deformities caused by relative shortening of muscles and soft tissues, and deformities of bones and joints, cannot be passively corrected. Fixed deformities must therefore be accommodated in orthoses or corrected by surgery to enable orthotic intervention. Intramuscular injections of botulinum A toxin are now commonly used as a way of temporarily weakening spastic muscles; during which time the range of motion at joints such as the ankle can be increased through serial casting or orthoses.

Ensuring muscles spend more than 6 hours in each 24-hour period in an elongated position may help to prevent or reduce the rate of progressive contractures (Tardieu et al. 1988). Solid ankle–foot orthoses (AFOs) are often prescribed for this purpose, for day or night use, in order to limit the progression of equinus deformity and knee gaiters are used to maintain the range of knee extended. However, it is suggested that stretching muscles using 'active forces' for shorter periods may be more effective to increase the range of motion at joints than orthoses that maintain the limb in a static position. Consequently there has been some preliminary research using orthoses incorporating components such as compressed gas pistons or coiled springs that generate active, usually extension, forces (Farmer et al. 2005).

To Provide a Base of Support

Stability in any position of lying, sitting or standing requires the centre of mass of the body to be positioned well with the supporting area. AFOs are often used to provide a stable base for standing and walking. Similarly, hip-abduction orthoses may improve sitting stability by increasing the size of the base of support.

To Facilitate Training in Skills

AFOs directly influence the alignment of the body segments supported within the device and, as described in the introductory chapters, they can also influence hip- and knee-joint moments by manipulating the direction of the ground reaction force. Stabilizing the ankle and foot therefore allows therapy to focus training on strengthening and encouraging better control over proximal joints. Other common training targets include encouraging better head control by providing trunk stability, and using wrist orthoses to facilitate manual dexterity when grasping objects. There may be a motor learning effect when children repeat movements (Butler et al. 1992).

To Improve the Efficiency of Gait

Children in GMFCS levels I–III, and to some extent those in level IV, should be encouraged to achieve an optimally efficient gait. Gage listed the prerequisites of normal gait first proposed by Perry (Gage 2004) which are summarized in Table 9.1. Lower-limb orthoses may improve gait efficiency by restoring these prerequisites through altering the forces acting on the body. Orthoses may also reduce energy expenditure further by decreasing the need for compensatory gait deviations to achieve locomotion.

Assessment

A thorough assessment of the individual child's needs is essential. The appropriate treatment plan for each child will be influenced by the severity of their impairments and their individual

TABLE 9.1
Prerequisites for efficient gait

Prerequisite	Qualifier
Stability of the stance limb	Requiring an appropriate foot floor contact area, minimizing the external moments acting on the knee and creating adequate hip abduction power to prevent the pelvis dropping on the unsupported side
Clearance of the swinging limb	Requiring adequate hip and knee flexion and ankle dorsiflexion of the swinging limb
Appropriate positioning of the limb at terminal swing	By knee extension and ankle dorsiflexion prior to initial stance contact
Achieving an adequate step length	By hip extension of the stance limb and unrestricted advancement of the swinging limb
Conservation of energy expenditure	Through reduced excursion of the centre of mass of the body

activity limitations and goals as well as their preferences and social circumstances. The effectiveness of any treatment will be influenced by the availability of physical therapy and the family's motivation. Assembling the relevant information for treatment planning is a multidisciplinary task involving not only an orthotist but also orthopaedic surgeons, developmental paediatricians, physiatrists, physical and occupational and speech and language therapists, social workers and others. The information will include a precise diagnosis, type and distribution of the impairment, functional motor status utilizing the GMFCS, ranges of joint motion passively and during activities, selective muscle control, strength, spasticity, joint congruency and integrity judged by imaging techniques such as X-ray or magnetic resonance imaging (MRI), plus details of any associated impairments. In addition, an assessment of sitting and standing balance and gait analysis may be required for children with those abilities. Another factor influencing assessment and the development of a realistic plan would be the various environments in which the child interacts.

Once the treatment goals are defined, many therapeutic interventions other than orthoses will be considered such as oral, intramuscular or intrathecally administered medications, orthopaedic and neurological surgery, physical and occupational therapy, wheelchairs, walking aids and other assistive technology, and temporary splinting and casting. These interventions may be prescribed to supplement and reduce the demands required of an orthosis and in some instances render the orthosis unnecessary. Whatever the treatment goals a family-centred approach will encourage compliance with the prescribed treatment regimen (King et al. 1999). The team must therefore be well coordinated, work in partnership with the family, provide adequate information about the condition, the role of interventions and their expected outcomes, and generally support the family (Rosenbaum et al. 1992). It is likely that therapy programmes that focus on practicing tasks that are important to the child and family are likely to improve functioning more than therapies that focus on normalising movement (Ketelaar et al. 2001). Although orthoses are prescribed for specific deformities or gait deviations, the level of each child's individual activity limitation will also influence the amount of support required; therefore the remainder of the chapter considers orthotic management with reference to the GMFCS.

GMFCS levels I, II and III

Approximately two-thirds of children with CP will achieve some level of walking ability (Pharoah et al. 1998). Children in GMFCS levels I, II and III learn to stand and walk later than unaffected children, and those in Level III are dependent on using assistive mobility aids. Examination will therefore include an assessment of the child's standing posture and gait. The gait of children with spastic cerebral palsy is generally repeatable from step to step; however the gait of children with ataxic or dyskinetic types are more variable. The difficulty in analysing the gait of children with cerebral palsy is that the impairment frequently causes deviations in the sagittal, coronal and transverse planes and may simultaneously involves the trunk, hips, knees and ankle joints. Instrumented three-dimensional gait analysis has vastly improved our understanding of the gait problems caused by cerebral palsy (Gage 2004).

Recommendations for orthotic intervention to improve gait efficiency are based on the integrity of the plantarflexion–knee extension couple. This describes the normal relationship between the ankle–foot complex and the knee joint to maintain the ground reaction force (GRF) just in front of the knee during stance phase. The foot must be leading approximately in the line of gait progression and the gastrocnemius and soleus muscles functioning eccentrically to control tibial advancement (Gage 2004).

SPASTIC HEMIPLEGIA

A comprehensive review of the management of hemiplegia is offered by Neville and Goodman (2000). Winters et al. (1987) classified sagittal plane gait abnormalities in children with hemiplegia into four distinct patterns with increasing distal to proximal pathology. Type I involves equinus only in swing phase, causing a foot clearance problem, which can be resolved using either a posterior leaf spring (PLS) (Fig. 9.3) or hinged AFO with a plantarflexion-stop. For type II hemiplegia, when equinus persists in both stance and swing phase and the knee tends towards hyperextension during stance, an appropriately tuned rigid AFO is recommended (Fig. 9.4). A hinged AFO with a plantarflexion-stop might be preferred by some prescribers providing there is a reasonable range of dorsiflexion with the knee extended. For Winters' types III and IV, when additional knee and hip involvement exists, orthotic management may help to resolve the foot and ankle problem but orthopaedic surgery is required to resolve the proximal impairments. The use of a knee gaiter to hold the knee extended may help to reduce the rate that a knee flexion deformity deteriorates.

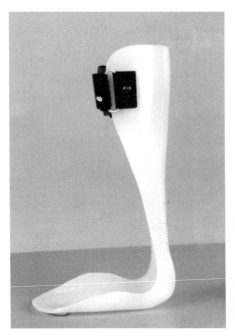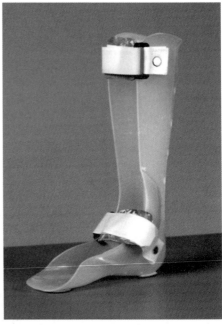

Fig. 9.3 Posterior leaf spring (PLS) AFO to prevent equinus in swing phase.

Fig. 9.4 A rigid AFO, designed to prevent equinus in stance and swing phases.

In addition to the sagittal-plane problems there can be a tendency for hindfoot varus if there is spasticity affecting the tibialis posterior muscle; this can be corrected in the AFO during the casting process and maintained with extra strapping if necessary. Winters' type IV hemiplegia can be associated with femoral anteversion causing an internal rotational foot-progression angle and some compensatory retraction of the pelvis on the affected side. Surgical correction of the anteversion leads to better function and a more symmetrical gait (Graham et al. 2005). Hip subluxation is rarely associated with hemiplegia (Soo et al. 2006).

As children with hemiplegia are predominantly classified in GMFCS levels I and II, they are by definition walking without mobility aids and perform most activities albeit slower and with qualitative differences. Provision of PLS or solid AFOs to prevent plantarflexion occasionally impede some tasks and the wearing regimen can be modified not to interfere with these activities; for instance the AFO might not usually be worn while participating in sports unless it improved the child's performance. Some children with hemiplegia have some control over their dorsiflexor muscles and experience such minor or no activity limitations that they prefer to not wear any AFO; or they may perhaps benefit from a foot orthosis to improve stability in stance.

Leg-length discrepancy (LLD) is often associated with hemiplegia but, as it is the weaker leg that is shorter, a small difference may be an advantage for achieving foot clearance in swing phase. Significant LLD causes pelvic obliquity in the coronal plane or compensatory excessive hip and knee flexion of the longer limb. Pelvic obliquity which results in hip adduction on the longer limb and hip abduction of the shorter side can be corrected using a shoe raise. An internal heel elevator or external shoe raise can then be used to fine tune the effect of the ground reaction force on the knee and hip joints, further enhancing gait efficiency. If necessary the LLD can be addressed surgically by epiphysiodesis to arrest growth in the longer limb at an appropriate age.

The upper limb is also affected in hemiplegia and a wrist hand orthosis (WHO) leaving the fingers and thumb free sometimes helps to improve function by holding the wrist in a functional position (Fig. 9.5); and a paddle-type design can be used to stretch the whole wrist and hand. A stiffened fabric gaiter can be used for short periods to stretch the elbow if flexion deformity occurs. There has been renewed interest in constraint-induced therapy to disable the good hand in an effort to encourage use of the impaired side (Eliasson et al. 2005, Naylor and Bower 2005).

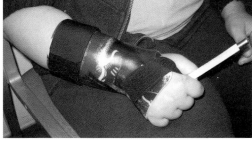

Fig. 9.5 Dorsal WHO with elastic Velcro straps worn by a child with hemiplegia to improve grasping.

Children with spastic diplegia commonly walk with the foot and ankle in equinus. Making initial contact with the forefoot during walking will usually cause the line of action of the ground reaction force (GRF) to pass in front of the knee joint and hip joint causing an excessive external knee extension moment, hyperextension (also called recurvatum or back-kneeing), and a flexion moment around the hip. Rigid AFOs that prevent plantarflexion and have been appropriately tuned can alter the direction of the GRF to reduce the resulting abnormal moments around the knee and hip joints, and prevent knee hyperextension and increase hip extension (Meadows 1984, Butler et al. 1992).

However, for children with more severe impairment, spasticity of proximal muscles will cause the knee and hip joints to remain flexed during stance (Gage 2004). When the GRF passes behind the knee the increased external flexion moment will cause excessive knee flexion and crouching. As a general rule the use of knee–ankle–foot orthoses (KAFOs) is not indicated for children with cerebral palsy. Anterior ground reaction AFOs that prevent dorsiflexion at the ankle can prevent knee flexion during stance by realigning the GRF in front of the knee (Saltiel 1969). However, whereas these orthoses are effective for paralysed limbs, as with myelomeningocoele, the presence of spastic or fixed-flexion deformities at the knee and hip means that these orthoses are ineffective without orthopaedic surgery to correct the proximal impairments (Harrington et al. 1983). The anterior ground reaction AFO is importantly employed following multilevel orthopaedic surgery to compensate for weakened calf and quadriceps muscle groups and promote an upright posture (Fig. 9.6).

In either of the above situations the rigid lever of the ankle and foot must also cope with premature and prolonged external dorsiflexion moment. The multisegmental structure of the

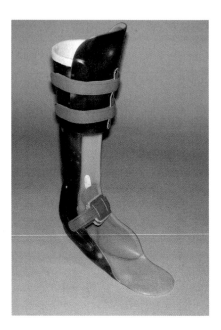

Fig. 9.6 Anterior ground reaction AFOs used following multilevel orthopaedic surgery compensate for quadriceps weakness and provide a stable base of support.

ankle and foot may buckle due the applied forces causing hindfoot eversion or inversion and midfoot collapse. In these circumstances apparent dorsiflexion will occur at the expense of the structure of the ankle and foot. Therefore when the integrity of the ankle and foot is insufficient to maintain a rigid lever, and the hindfoot and midfoot are at risk of deformity, it may be as important to prevent dorsiflexion as well as plantarflexion using a rigid AFO.

Sutherland and Davids (1993) identified four patterns of knee motion in children with spastic diplegia based on sagittal-plane kinematics, namely jump knee, crouch knee, stiff knee and recurvatum knee. In combination with Winters' classification, these patterns have been used to create algorithms for physical management combining various interventions including recommendations for orthoses (Rodda et al. 2004). The systems used to classify gait should however be used judiciously as there are major limitations of their validity and reliability (Dobson et al. 2006a, b).

Pelvic rotation, torsional abnormalities or foot deformities can change the angle of the foot in relation to the line of progression (in- or out-toeing). However, gait deviations in the coronal and transverse planes are more difficult to distinguish than those in the sagittal plane using only observational gait analysis. 'Apparent' rather than true hip adduction occurs when internal rotation is seen simultaneously with hip flexion causing the knees to come together when viewed in the coronal plane (sometimes called 'scissor' gait). Femoral anteversion occurs frequently in children with CP because of their delayed motor milestones in standing and walking and for ambulant children is more common than true hip adduction. Hip-abduction orthoses for ambulant children may therefore be of little benefit other than to hold the knees apart.

Although it may be possible to harness shear forces from the skin and the shape of the soft tissues to gain some rotational control using a moulded thigh cuff, in general rotational control of the hip joint using orthoses requires extension to the foot.

Twister orthoses incorporating a flexible torque cable extending from a waistband to an AFO or elastic fabric wound around the limb attached to AFOs create active rotational forces and can alter the foot-progression angle (Nuzzo 1980). However, when the cause of internal hip rotation is persistent femoral anteversion or spasticity, as more often is the case, twister orthoses are little more than temporary solutions; they may increase spasticity, and the restrictions imposed by such orthoses may therefore not justify their use. Torsional lower-limb deformities usually require femoral osteotomy which also improves the efficiency of hip-abductor muscles by increasing the length of their leverage. However, as the surgery is not performed until the child is aged 6–8 years, twister orthoses can be useful in the short term as an adjunct to multilevel botulinum toxin injections. In- or out-toeing may also result from excessive pelvic rotation or foot deformity when there may be no torsional component in the long bones. Mobile deformities of hindfoot inversion with associated forefoot adduction, and hindfoot eversion with associated forefoot abduction, can be corrected during the casting process and controlled using AFOs.

Many studies have attempted to compare the efficacy of rigid, hinged, PLS AFOs and supramalleolar foot orthoses. A review of the efficacy of orthoses for children with CP including 28 studies and more than 450 children concluded that preventing plantarflexion improved gait efficiency (Morris 2002). Preventing plantarflexion has been shown to improve stability in stance phase (Miller and Chambers 1998–1999), clearance in swing phase (Õunpuu et al. 1996), pre-positioning in terminal swing (Romskes and Brunner 2000), and increase step length and walking speed (Abel et al. 1998). There is a suggestion that preventing plantarflexion also improves energy expenditure based on oxygen consumption (Maltais et al. 2001). There is no evidence to support any tone reducing effect on gait from orthoses that incorporate specially moulded footplates (Crenshaw et al. 2000).

GMFCS levels IV and V

Children in GMFCS levels IV and V might be classified as having spastic diplegia or quadriplegia and are more severely limited in their activities. AFOs are used to limit equinus deformity and to provide a stable base and encourage weight-bearing during standing transfers. Maintaining reasonable foot and ankle posture will enable more comfortable posture in seating systems by allowing some of the weight of the lower limbs to be supported by footplates. If profound fixed ankle and foot deformities become established then fitting of ordinary shoes can become a problem and custom-made footwear or surgical treatment may be required. Children at level V spend all their time in either lying or sitting postures. They are therefore dependent on the provision of appropriate seating and lying postural management systems for comfort and optimal functioning. The provision of these forms of assistive technology must be planned in conjunction with orthotic management. In addition to limb deformities, children at GMFCS levels IV and V are susceptible to developing scoliosis and hip subluxation/dislocation.

Scoliosis

Children in GMFCS levels IV and V are at greater risk of scoliosis (Fig. 9.7), which appears to be aggravated by the effects of gravity when the individuals were placed in the sitting position (Madigan and Wallace 1981). Rigid plastic thoracolumbar sacral orthoses (TLSOs) may reduce spinal curvature and improve sitting ability whilst the orthosis is worn (Terjesen et al. 2000), but TLSOs are unlikely to alter the rate of progressive deformity (Miller et al. 1996). For children with large structural scoliosis surgical stabilization will be the more realistic intervention to offer the child and family. A child using a TLSO in conjunction with a modular seating system is shown in Figure 9.8.

When casting for spinal orthoses it is preferable to remove the deforming effect of gravity; however, as the treatment goal will be to enable a comfortable and functional sitting posture, overcorrection may not be indicated. Tight hamstrings, as demonstrated by a reduced popliteal angle, can reduce the lumbar lordosis by posteriorly tilting the pelvis (sometimes called sacral sitting) and, at times, hamstring lengthening can help to improve sitting posture. Children with poor levels of sitting ability may also demonstrate excessive forward trunk leaning or thoracic kyphosis. Spinal orthoses may prevent forward leaning and one study has suggested that the improved positioning achieved with a spinal orthosis may improve pulmonary functioning (Leopando et al. 1999).

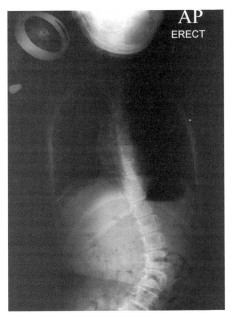

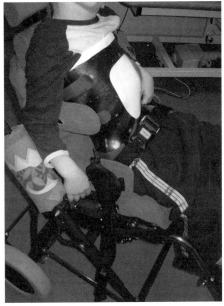

Fig. 9.7 Characteristic *long-C* pattern of scoliosis sometimes seen in children with cerebral palsy in GMFCS levels IV and V.

Fig. 9.8 Example of a TLSO for a child with cerebral palsy GMFCS level V, the orthosis is being used in combination with a modular seating system to provide postural support.

HIP SUBLUXATION

Hip subluxation and dislocation is caused by muscle imbalance around the joint and is highly associated with the severity of impairment. The risk of hip displacement of 30% or greater was 4–6 times more for children in GMFCS levels IV and V than level I and II (Soo et al. 2006). Hip dislocation requiring treatment before age 5 years was observed more commonly in children with spastic cerebral palsy who were non-ambulant compared with those who could walk 10 steps by age 30 months (Scrutton et al. 2001). The hip is particularly at risk of dislocation when the range of passive hip abduction (in flexion) reduces below 45°. Hip deformity can be classified as symmetrical or asymmetrical and the latter often described as windswept deformity.

Orthoses can theoretically be used to increase containment of the femoral head in the acetabulum, by abducting and flexing the hip joint, and also stretching the adductor muscles to maintain the range of abduction to greater than 45°. This is occasionally undertaken in conjunction with neurolytic agents or botulinum A toxin to weaken the spastic muscles causing subluxation. There have been claims that a regimen incorporating the standing, walking and sitting hip-abduction (SWASH) orthosis with regular botulinum A toxin injections reduces the need for surgery (Boyd et al. 2001, 2003); however, longer follow-up suggests that the need for surgery is merely delayed with little benefit (Graham and Selber 2006). This seems to support the assertions by Hagglund (2005) that hip dislocation can only be ameliorated by early surgery, and orthotic intervention has limited benefit. Surgery to reconstruct of the hip may be considered if hip subluxation becomes painful and orthoses may play a part in the postoperative regimen. The most versatile hip orthosis (HpO) for use in the postoperative period includes an orthotic hip hinge that allows incremental adjustment of flexion and abduction and can be locked in the selected position. Alternatively, a total body splint made from low-temperature plastics can be used to maintain the hip abducted. There are proprietary lying and sleeping orthoses that can be used as part of a 24-hour postural management regimen (Pountney and Green 2006); this may provide comfort but it is unclear whether there is any effect on preventing deformity developing over time.

Abducting the hips to increase the size of the base of support can have the functional benefit of improving sitting stability. For non-ambulant children, the benefits of the TLSO in controlling the position of the centre of gravity and stabilizing the trunk as a single segment can be combined with hip-abduction orthosis providing a stable base in a hip-abduction spinal sitting orthoses (HASSOs) (Drake and Boyd 1993); however, this is more usually achieved using customized seating systems.

Summary

This chapter has utilised the GMFCS as an ability-based framework for distinguishing treatment goals for orthotic management for children with cerebral palsy. Owing to the complexity of the manifestations of cerebral palsy and the varying backgrounds and beliefs of professionals there is variation in orthoses recommended by different health professionals. A trend in the 1990s for so-called 'tone-reducing' AFOs, which incorporate specially shaped footplates, seems to have dissipated and it is evident that orthoses predominantly work through biomechanical effects. Some orthoses can seem bulky and an encumbrance; however such orthoses often help to prevent deformities and improve the functioning of children with cerebral palsy.

References

Abel MF, Juhl GA, Vaughan CL, Damiano DL (1998) Gait assessment of fixed ankle–foot orthoses in children with spastic diplegia. *Arch Phys Med Rehabil* **79**: 126–33.
Boyd R, Graham H, Natrass G, Reddihough D, Thomason P, Homason P, Dobson F, Parrott J, Lowe K, Lancaster A (2003) Botulinum toxin A (BTX-A) combined with hip bracing delays the need for surgery in children with bilateral cerebral palsy: a randomized clinical trial and survivorship analysis (abstract). *Dev Med Child Neurol* **45** (suppl. 96): 10.
Boyd RN, Dobson F, Parrott J, Love S, Oates J, Larson A, Burchall G, Chondros P, Carlin J, Nattrass G, Graham HK (2001) The effect of botulinum toxin type A and a variable hip abduction orthosis on gross motor function: a randomized controlled trial. *Eur J Neurol* **8** (suppl. 5): 109–19.
Butler PB, Thompson N, Major RE (1992) Improvement in walking performance of children with cerebral palsy: preliminary results. *Dev Med Child Neurol* **34**: 567–76.
Condie DN, Meadows CB (1995) *Report of a Consensus Conference on the Lower Limb Orthotic Management of Cerebral Palsy*. Copenhagen: International Society of Prosthetics & Orthotics.
Crenshaw S, Herzog R, Castagno P, Richards J, Miller F, Michaloski G, Moran E (2000) The efficacy of tone-reducing features in orthotics on the gait of children with spastic diplegic cerebral palsy. *J Pediatr Orthop* **20**: 210–16.
Dobson F, Morris ME, Baker R, Graham HK (2006a) Gait classification in children with cerebral palsy: a systematic review. *Gait Posture* **25**: 140–52.

Dobson F, Morris M, Baker R, Wolfe R, Graham H (2006b) Clinician agreement on gait pattern ratings in children with spastic hemiplegia. *Dev Med Child Neurol* **48**: 429–35.

Drake C, Boyd R (1993) The design and manufacture of a thermoplastic hip abduction and spinal orthosis for bilateral non ambulant cerebral palsy children. *ISPO UK Newsletter* Summer, 25–6.

Eliasson AC, Krumlinde-Sundholm L, Shaw K, Wang C (2005) Effects of constraint-induced movement therapy in young children with hemiplegic cerebral palsy: an adapted model. *Dev Med Child Neurol* **47**: 266–75.

Farmer SE, Woollam PJ, Patrick JH, Roberts AP, Bromwich W (2005) Dynamic orthoses in the management of joint contracture. *J Bone Joint Surg Br* **87**: 291–5.

Gage JR (2004) *The Treatment of Gait Problems in Cerebral Palsy*. London: Mac Keith Press.

Graham HK (2002) Painful hip dislocation in cerebral palsy. *Lancet* **359**: 907 –8.

Graham HK, Harvey A, Rodda J, Nattrass GR, Pirpiris M (2004) The Functional Mobility Scale (FMS). *J Pediatr Orthop* **24**: 514–20.

Graham HK, Baker R, Dobson F, Morris ME (2005) Multilevel orthopaedic surgery in group IV spastic hemiplegia. *J Bone Joint Surg Br* **87**: 548–55.

Graham HK, Selber P (2006) After the randomized clinical trial was over: longer term follow-up of children with cerebral palsy after participation in a randomized clinical trial of non-operative management of hip in displacement. *Dev Med Child Neurol* **48** (Suppl. 105): 7–8.

Hagglund G, Andersson S, Duppe H, Lauge-Pedersen H, Nordmark E, Westbom L (2005) Prevention of dislocation of the hip in children with cerebral palsy. The first ten years of a population-based prevention programme. *J Bone Joint Surg* **87**: 95–101.

Harrington ED, Lin RS, Gage JR (1983) Use of the anterior floor reaction orthosis in patients with cerebral palsy. *Orthot Prosthet* **37**: 34–42.

Kennes J, Rosenbaum P, Hanna SE, Walter S, Russell D, Raina P, Bartlett D, Galuppi B (2002) Health status of school-aged children with cerebral palsy: information from a population-based sample. *Dev Med Child Neurol* **44**: 240–7.

Ketelaar M, Vermeer A, Hart H, van Petegem-van Beek E, Helders PJ (2001) Effects of a functional therapy program on motor abilities of children with cerebral palsy. *Phys Ther* **81**: 1534–45.

King G, King S, Rosenbaum P, Goffin R (1999) Family-centered caregiving and well-being of parents of children with disabilities: linking process with outcomes. *J Pediatr Psychol* **24**: 41–53.

Leopando MT, Moussavi Z, Holbrow J, Chernick V, Pasterkamp H, Rempel G (1999) Effect of a Soft Boston Orthosis on pulmonary mechanics in severe cerebral palsy. *Pediatr Pulmon* **28**: 53–8.

Madigan RR, Wallace SL (1981) Scoliosis in the institutionalized cerebral palsy population. *Spine* **6**: 583–90.

Maltais D, Bar-Or O, Galea V, Pierrynowski M (2001) Use of orthoses lowers the O_2 cost of walking in children with spastic cerebral palsy. *Med Science Sports Exerc* **33**: 320–5.

Meadows CB (1984) *The influence of polypropylene ankle-foot orthoses on the gait of cerebral palsied children*. PhD thesis, University of Strathclyde.

Miller A, Temple T, Miller F (1996) Impact of orthoses on the rate of scoliosis progression in children with cerebral palsy *J Pediatr Orthop* **16**: 332–5.

Miller NH, Chambers C (1998–1999) Dynamic versus standard AFOs: a comparison of gait parameters (abstract). *Orthopaedic Trans* **22**: 452.

Morris C (2002) A Review of the efficacy of lower limb orthoses used for cerebral palsy. *Dev Med Child Neurol* **44**: 205–11.

Morris C, Newdick H, Johnson A (2002) Variations in the orthotic management of cerebral palsy. *Child: Care Health Dev* **28**: 139–47.

Morris, C. Bartlett, D. (2004) Gross Motor Function Classification System: impact and utility. *Dev Med Child Neurol* **46**: 60–5.

Neville B, Goodman R. (2000) *Congenital Hemiplegia*. London: Mac Keith Press.

Naylor CE, Bower E (2005) Modified constraint-induced movement therapy for young children with hemiplegic cerebral palsy: a pilot study. *Dev Med Child Neurol* **47**: 365–9.

Nuzzo RM (1980) Dynamic bracing: elastics for patients with cerebral palsy, muscular dystrophy and myelodysplasia. *Clin Orthop* **148**: 263–73.

Õunpuu S, Bell KJ, Davis RB 3, DeLuca PA (1996) An evaluation of the posterior leaf spring orthosis using joint kinematics and kinetics. *J Pediatr Orthop* **16**: 378–84.

Palisano R, Rosenbaum P, Walter S, Russell D, Wood E, Galuppi B (1997) Development and reliability of a system to classify gross motor function in children with cerebral palsy. *Dev Med Child Neurol* **39**: 214–23.

Pharoah PO, Cooke T, Johnson MA, King R, Mutch L (1998) Epidemiology of cerebral palsy in England and Scotland, 1984–9. *Arch Dis Child, Fetal & Neonat Edn* **79**: F21–5.

99

Pountney T, Green EM (2006) Hip dislocation in cerebral palsy. *BMJ* **332**: 772–5.

Rodda J, Graham HK, Carson L, Galea MP, Wolfe R (2004) Sagittal gait patterns in spastic diplegia. *J Bone Joint Surg Br* **86**: 251–8.

Romskes J, Brunner R (2002) Comparison of a dynamic and a hinged ankle-foot orthosis by gait analysis in patients with hemiplegic cerebral palsy *Gait Posture* **15**: 18–24.

Russell DJ, Gorter JW (2005) Assessing functional differences in gross motor skills in children with cerebral palsy who use and ambulatory aid or orthoses: can the GMFM-88 help? *Dev Med Child Neurol* **47**: 462–7.

Rosenbaum PL, King SM, Cadman DT (1992) Measuring processes of caregiving to physically disabled children and their families. 1: Identifying relevant components of care. *Dev Med Child Neurol* **34**: 103–14.

Rosenbaum PL, Walter SD, Hanna SE, Palisano RJ, Russell DJ, Raina P, Wood E, Bartlett DJ, Galuppi BE (2002) Prognosis for gross motor function in cerebral palsy creation of motor development curves. *JAMA* **288**: 1357–63.

Rosenbaum PL, Paneth N, Leviton A, Goldsteini M, Bax M, Damiano D, Dan B, Jacobsson B (2007) A report: the definition and classification of cerebral palsy, April 2006. *Dev Med Child Neurol* **109** (suppl.) 8–14.

Saltiel J (1969) A one-piece laminated knee locking short leg brace. *Orthot Prosthet* **23**: 68–75.

Scrutton, D., Baird, G. Smeeton, N. (2001) Hip dysplasia in bilateral cerebral palsy: incidence and natural history in children aged 18 months to 5 years. *Dev Med Child Neurol* **43**: 586–600.

Soo B, Howard JJ, Boyd RN, Reid SM, Lanigan A, Wolfe R, Reddihough D, Graham HK (2006) Hip displacement in cerebral palsy. *J Bone Joint Surg Am* **88**: 121–9.

Surveillance of Cerebral Palsy in Europe (SCPE) (2000) Surveillance of cerebral palsy in Europe: a collaboration of cerebral palsy surveys and registers. *Dev Med Child Neurol* **42**: 816–24.

Sutherland, D.H. Davids, J.R. (1993) Common gait abnormalities of the knee in cerebral palsy. *Clin Orthop* **288**: 139–47.

Tardieu C, Lespargot A, Tabary C, Bret MD (1988) For how long must the soleus muscle be stretched each day to prevent contracture? *Dev Med and Child Neurol* **30**: 3–10.

Terjesen T, Lange JE, Steen H (2000) Treatment of scoliosis with spinal bracing in quadriplegic cerebral palsy. *Dev Med Child Neurol* **42**: 448–54.

Winters TFJr, Gage JR, Hicks R (1987) Gait patterns in spastic hemiplegia in children and young adults. *J Bone Joint Surg Am* **69**: 437–41.

Vos-Vromans DC, Ketelaar M, Gorter JW (2005) Responsiveness of evaluative measures for children with cerebral palsy: the Gross Motor Function Measure and the Pediatric Evaluation of Disability Inventory. *Disab Rehabil* **27**: 1245–52.

Ziv I, Blackburn N, Rang M, Koreska J. (1984) Muscle growth in normal and spastic mice. *Dev Med Child Neurol* **26**: 94–9.

10
MUSCULAR DYSTROPHIES, SPINAL MUSCULAR ATROPHIES AND PERIPHERAL NEUROPATHIES

Nicola Thompson, Stephen Porter and Christopher Morris

Neuromuscular diseases considered in this chapter are inherited disorders which often lead to significant physical disability and, in some conditions, reduced life expectancy. The conditions can be broadly subdivided into two groups: (1) myopathies, where the pathology is confined to the muscle, for example Duchenne muscular dystrophy (DMD); and (2) neuropathies, where the primary problem occurs in the peripheral nerves causing secondary impairment of the muscles, for example hereditary motor sensory neuropathies (HMSN) (Table 10.1). These disorders are also generally classified by the genetic defect. This chapter describes aspects of orthotic management that may be helpful in the physical management of children with the more common disorders.

Muscle weakness is the primary feature of all these neuromuscular diseases while the degree and distribution of weakness varies between conditions. The weakness is commonly associated with joint contractures and deformities, which may also in turn further compromise motor and/or respiratory functions. Muscle diseases can be either progressive or non-progressive, but in the growing child increasing height and weight may also contribute to loss of function and an apparent deterioration. For more comprehensive details regarding the diagnosis, prognosis and general management the reader is referred to Dubowitz (1995). The physical management of children affected by these conditions requires an integrated multidisciplinary approach; the orthotic treatment objectives include:

- to maintain/improve muscle strength
- to control/prevent joint contractures
- to maximize motor function
- to control scoliosis
- to preserve respiratory function.

The muscular dystrophies are a group of genetically determined disorders associated with progressive degeneration of skeletal muscle. They can be subdivided into a number of different disorders based upon the mode of inheritance, protein, enzyme and/or genetic defect as well as the degree and distribution of muscle weakness. The Xp21.2 myopathies

TABLE 10.1.
**Classification of neuromuscular diseases according to the site of
defect in the motor unit (after Thompson and Quinlivan 2004)**

Site of defect	Diagnosis
Anterior horn cell	Spinal muscular atrophy (SMA) (proximal and distal) Poliomyelitis Motor neurone disease (involves the motor unit & upper motorneurones)
Nerve fibre	Hereditary motor sensory neuropathies (HMSN) Inflammatory neuropathies, e.g. chronic inflammatory demyelinating polyradiculopathy, CIDP) Toxic neuropathy (e.g. organophosphates, mercury) Metabolic neuropathy (e.g. metachromatic leucodystrophy, Refsum's disease)
Neuromuscular junction	Myasthenia gravis Congenital myathenic syndromes Lambert–Eaton syndrome
Muscle fibre	Congenital myopathies, e.g. central core disease Collagen disorders (Bethlem myopathy) Mitochondrial myopathies Glycogen storage diseases affecting muscle (e.g. acid maltese deficiency, McArdle's disease) Disorders of lipid metabolism and fatty acid Oxidation (eg carnitine and CPT11 deficiencies) Inflammatory myopathies (eg polymyositis, dermatomyositis and inclusion body myositis) Endocrine myopathies (thyroid dysfunction and hyperparathyroidism) Muscle channelopathies (e.g. sodium channel and muscle chloride channel diseases

or dystrophinopathies are progressive muscle disorders that include the rapidly progressive DMD and the more mildly progressive, though nonetheless disabling, Becker muscular dystrophy (BMD). They are caused by a defect of the protein dystrophin which is normally present on the surface membrane of muscle and also found in the brain, resulting in muscle degeneration and eventual replacement by fat and connective tissue. They are characterized by X-linked inheritance, in which males are affected and females are carriers: spontaneous mutation is also possible.

Duchenne muscular dystrophy
The initial manifestations of DMD appear when a child shows slightly delayed motor milestones at 3–5 years. Physical examination reveals proximal muscle weakness causing limitations in the activities of running, jumping and climbing stairs. The natural history is characterized by progressive weakness affecting proximal muscles earlier than those more distal. This leads to compensatory postural abnormalities such as hyperlordosis and equinus, the development of muscle contractures, and a relentless increase in the effort in walking. Gowers' manoeuvre describes the characteristic way in which boys use their upper limb

strength to climb up their legs when getting up from the floor in order to compensate for weakness of the hip- and knee-extensors (Gowers 1879). Muscle enlargement, most commonly in the calves, is due to an excess of adipose and connective tissue and therefore the term pseudohypertrophy is used. The boys become totally dependent on a wheelchair for mobility by the age of 12 years. The later period of wheelchair dependence is accompanied by a rapid increase in limb joint contractures and progressive spinal deformity. Approximately two-thirds of boys affected by DMD have below-average intelligence (Dubowitz 1995).

Despite the rather grim prognosis a significant improvement in the quality and duration of life can be made by maximizing the care provided to the boys and family. A variety of orthotic, therapeutic and surgical measures are available that can help minimize deformity, prolong independent ambulation and maximize functional capabilities (Galasko et al. 1992, Vignos et al. 1996). Most boys die from respiratory or cardiac failure, but the introduction of nocturnal nasal ventilation has improved survival, such that the average life expectancy is now 25 years with non-invasive ventilation, compared with 19 years without this treatment (Eagle et al. 2002). From an orthotic management perspective the course of DMD may be divided into three phases: early ambulatory, late ambulatory and non-ambulatory.

EARLY AMBULATORY PHASE

Joint contractures compromise the efficiency of weakened muscles and further impair mobility and function. Contractures develop due to a combination of muscle strength imbalance across joints and gradual fibrosis within the muscles. Certain patterns develop consistently, such as hip-flexor and iliotibial band tightness secondary to pelvic girdle weakness. The larger hip- and knee-extensor muscles are key groups associated with early functional decline and deteriorating gait. Equinus or equinovarus deformities develop partially due to relative weakness of the anterior tibial and peroneal muscles but primarily as a compensation for quadriceps weakness. Instrumented motion analysis has revealed that the ankle equinus is assumed during gait to keep the ground reaction force anterior to the knee joint during stance phase, thereby maintaining stability (Sutherland et al. 1981, Khodadadeh et al. 1986). Consequently, the shortened calf muscles which typically accompany disease progression are often secondary to this necessary compensation during gait rather than due solely to the primary pathology.

For this reason, whilst the child remains independently ambulant, providing ankle–foot orthoses (AFOs) to correct toe-walking is likely to be detrimental to the child's mobility as will interfere with the compensatory mechanism described above and AFOs to reduce equinus should be confined to night use only. In many boys the foot appears excessively pronated as the medial arch is compromised by the reduced length of the calf muscles; there is therefore no indication to prescribe foot orthoses. A combination of passive stretching exercises and use of night AFOs is more effective than passive stretching alone in delaying contractures and prolonging independent ambulation (Scott et al. 1981, Hyde et al. 2000). Night AFOs should be offered when the child shows signs of toe walking and/or the range of passive ankle dorsiflexion with the knee extended is reduced. Given that these AFOs will be used predominantly at night they can be made either from polythene or thin (3 mm) polypropylene. The ankle posture should be easily tolerated by the child so not to interfere with sleep, usually just plantargrade or only very slightly dorsiflexed. The plastic might be better hand-draped rather than vacuum formed to create a looser fit around the leg section, especially bearing in mind the tendency for pseudohypertrophy. The foot-piece must be full length to provide adequate leverage to prevent equinus and allow for growth. There is little indication for padding inside the AFO throughout, however padding should be incorporated over the malleoli and perhaps the backs of the heels which often become tender; this padding can be added to the cast prior to moulding so that the inside of the AFO is smooth. One wide and well padded heel retaining strap is usually sufficient to contain the foot and ankle in the desired position and a calf strap is added to hold the AFO in place on the leg (Fig. 10.1).

LATE AMBULATORY PHASE

The aim of physical management is to prolong independent ambulation for as long as possible, since scoliosis and joint contractures develop rapidly once the ability to stand and

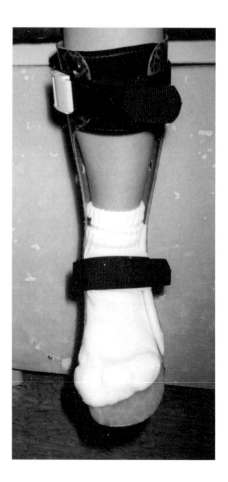

Fig. 10.1 Typical night AFO for boy with DMD.

walk is lost. In 1962 Spencer and Vignos first described a programme of heel-cord tenotomy and rehabilitation in knee–ankle–foot orthoses (KAFOs) to extend the independent walking ability of boys with DMD. This approach is now widely used as a means of prolonging mobility after independent walking ceases (see Fig. 10.5a, b) and has been shown to impede the long-term development of both lower limb contractures (Vignos et al. 1996) and scoliosis (Rodillo et al. 1988). Surgery may not always be required to correct the equinus, particularly if a programme of night AFOs has been used. However, to ensure the best chance of success, when surgery is necessary it is crucial that the KAFOs are ready immediately after the operation and that fitting problems are resolved expediently. The boys walk with an increased lumbar lordosis to maintain their balance due to tightness of the hip-flexor and weakness of hip-extensor muscles; they also use excessive trunk side flexion to compensate for hip-abductor weakness. This combination of hyperlordotic posture and exaggerated trunk movement is thought to help protect against the development of scoliosis. Gains in additional walking time vary among children and reported by different centres, but between 18 months to 4 years of walking can be achieved (Bakker et al. 2000).

John Florence was an orthotist (now retired) who specialized in paediatric orthotics and worked for many years at what is now called the Dubowitz Neuromuscular Centre, London, UK. During this time he developed several orthoses that are particularly suited for meeting the needs of children with muscle weakness. One of these components is the anterior Chailey lever which incorporates a 'cam' system for unlocking the orthotic knee hinges with less effort, even when the orthosis is under load (Fig. 10.2). The hinge can be unlocked easily by the boys or their carers as the lever is large and the mechanism simple to operate, even with limited dexterity and strength. The hinge is commercially available with either steel or aluminium side members although where possible aluminium should be preferred in order to minimize the overall weight of the orthosis. For boys with DMD the hinge is incorporated into polypropylene ischial bearing KAFOs. Using a two-stage casting process helps to ensure symmetry of the KAFOs; the ankles are cast first at a right angle with the child sitting up, then the child lies down while the cast is extended to the ischium and groin (Fig. 10.3a, b). When measuring for KAFOs prior to surgery for equinus, the foot angle must be corrected in the cast prior to filling the positive cast, to mimic the result of the expected surgical correction.

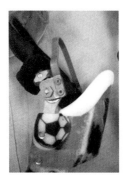

Fig. 10.2 Chailey knee hinge which incorporates a cam mechanism to making unlocking easier.

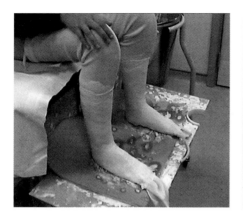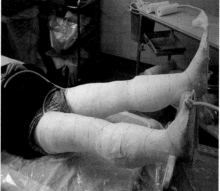

Fig. 10.3 A two-stage casting process when measuring for KAFOs helps to ensures that the ankle postures are symmetrical.

Polypropylene is hand-draped over the prepared positive cast and shaped side members. The thigh section includes a flared lip that is fits under the ischium. The AFO section is a solid ankle design and the foot-piece extends to 10–20 mm behind the metatarsal heads. This enables the boys to use their toe-flexors to aid balance and for the heel to rise as they walk forward. Once the posterior sections are trimmed the anterior plastic sections are moulded over 6 mm padding material, and riveted to the below-knee section (Fig. 10.4). This gives excellent control of the knees even with mild knee-flexion contractures and ensures symmetrical extension of the legs that may not be assured using other means of fastening. The calf and thigh sections are attached to the metal side members with screws to allow adjustment of length and flexion during growth.

At the initial fitting the orthotist should ensure that the height of the proximal lip of the thigh section is bearing sufficiently high into the under the buttocks (Fig. 10.5); whilst also ensuring that there is sufficient clearance in the groin area. Sometimes small heel raises are required inside the footwear to help the child attain standing balance. Once independent

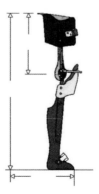

Fig. 10.4 John Florence design of KAFO.

106

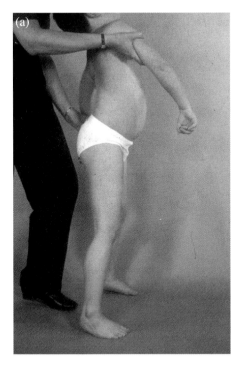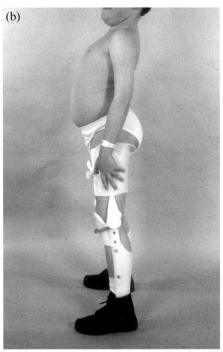

Fig. 10.5 (a) A boy with DMD at point of loss of ambulation, and (b) following tendo-Achilles tenotomies and rehabilitation in KAFOs.

standing is achieved the boys need to learn how to walk in the KAFOs. They must develop pelvic control to shift weight onto the stance limb and then use increased lateral flexion of the trunk to aid clearance of the swing limb – this will result in a side-to-side rocking action to move forward. Mobility aids are not necessary and in fact impede the adapted gait by encouraging forward trunk lean – instructing the boys to tuck their thumbs into the tops of the thigh sections can help to maintain an adequate lumbar lordosis and aid balance. Lightweight sports style footwear is the preferred type of footwear with a wedged non-slip sole. Cotton stocking or other material may need to be used as an interface between the plastic and the child's leg to prevent any discomfort caused by perspiration.

Selecting the appropriate time for intervention is crucial to the success of prolonging ambulation. The optimal time for providing the orthoses is when the child has lost independent walking but is still able to stand or walk a few steps with help (Fig. 10.5a). However, once the child has been wheelchair-bound for even a short time fixed lower limb deformities and muscle weakness rapidly progress, so any delay in undertaking this programme may compromise a successful outcome. Therefore only a small window of opportunity occurs in which the boys can benefit from KAFOs and this might be missed if follow-up appointments are too infrequent. Two factors which help to predict a successful outcome are the absence of severe hip and knee contractures and the percentage of residual muscle strength

(Hyde et al. 1982). The parents and child must also be strongly motivated as considerable effort and commitment is required. Not every child is appropriate for rehabilitation in KAFOs or simply may not wish to pursue this mode of treatment; some boys are afraid of falling over which is a risk although, in our experience, an extremely rare occurrence. A standing frame is an alternative option that enables safe standing as an activity as well as being potentially beneficial in terms of controlling lower-limb contractures and reducing the rate of scoliosis progression.

There is increasing evidence of the benefits of corticosteroid treatment in Duchenne muscular dystrophy. In recent reviews of steroid trials (Manzur et al. 2004, Moxley et al. 2005) the use of steroids has resulted in short-term improvements in muscle strength and function as well as a significant slowing of the progression of weakness. One small study used prolongation of walking (without KAFOs) as an outcome measure but did not show significant benefit. Close monitoring of side effects is required which includes excessive weight gain and behavioural abnormalities. Dosages can be lowered and still result in significant but less robust improvements. On the basis on the randomized trials published to date it is not yet possible to evaluate the long-term benefits and hazards of treatment using steroids.

NON-AMBULATORY PHASE
When the boys become wheelchair-dependent then a transition from night to daytime use of AFOs is recommended in an effort to prevent progressive foot deformity. Difficulty with wearing shoes and discomfort can result when equinovarus deformities become established; maintaining the feet in a plantargrade position may also assist the carer in transfers when hoists etc are unavailable. Where a varus hindfoot deformity is present the use of a lateral Y-strap lined with a soft material should be used instead of a heel strap (Fig. 10.6). However, the most pressing issues now concern achieving a comfortable sitting posture and monitoring any spinal deformity.

Whilst scoliosis is also associated with other neuromuscular disorders, it is markedly more progressive in boys with DMD due to the combination of increasing muscle weakness, rapid growth and gravity. The deformity becomes apparent as walking is increasingly limited and deteriorates rapidly once the child becomes dependent on a wheelchair. The curve usually develops as a paralytic 'long C' pattern in the thoracolumbar region and is often associated with pelvic obliquity. Spinal deformity can further compromise respiratory

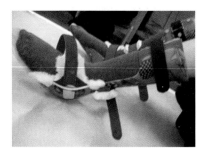

Fig. 10.6 AFO with extra Y-strap to correct hindfoot varus.

capacity, which is already restricted by the impaired respiratory muscle. Increasing scoliosis also leads to difficulty in sitting comfortably and maintaining head control. Depending on the child's and family's preferences, cardiopulmonary function and skeletal maturity the scoliosis can be managed either conservatively using a spinal orthosis or by surgical stabilization. Surgery needs to be considered early as the deformity is then likely to be amenable to correction and cardiopulmonary function is still adequate so the boys are better able to cope with the long procedure; cardiac and respiratory tests will precede any surgery to ensure they are sufficiently fit to undergo the procedure. Spinal instrumentation provides rigid internal fixation and obviates the need for postoperative immobilization or orthoses.

The spine should be monitored carefully in conjunction with the respiratory capacity. Prompt provision of a spinal orthosis is advisable when the curve is approximately 30°, and is only worn during the day whilst the child is upright. The orthosis should be as corrective as possible rather than simply supportive and this can be confirmed by comparing Cobb's angle from radiographs with and without the spinal orthosis. It is recognized that spinal bracing is not the definitive treatment in curves that are known to be rapidly progressive, but it is important in slowing the rate of progression of the curvature (Seeger et al. 1990). Spinal orthoses can be used with children who are unsuitable for surgery or choose to decline the procedure, and for children in whom fusion is not yet indicated. Close monitoring continues whilst the child is wearing a spinal orthosis, so that spinal surgery can be offered before cardiopulmonary function deteriorates to a point where anaesthesia presents an unacceptably high risk. Spinal bracing in a child with established severe scoliosis may cause appreciable respiratory impairment when there is respiratory muscle involvement, and is less likely to be tolerated than early prophylactic bracing (Noble-Jamieson et al. 1986).

The aim of orthotic management is to combine maximum correction of a scoliosis with maximum patient comfort and compliance, although these are not always easy to reconcile. A rigid material such as polypropylene is likely to provide the greatest correction, whilst more flexible and softer materials might be more comfortable but provide less support. Another option is to reinforce a jacket made from foamed polyethylene or one of the flexible materials particularly for severe deformity. Three designs of thoracolumbar spinal orthosis (TLSO) are likely to be appropriate: (1) a wraparound one-piece jacket, (2) separate back and front sections, or (3) separate side sections (Figs 10.7–10.9). The one-piece design is the easiest to make, is the least bulky and probably provides the best control of the spine. The front and back bivalve design makes it slightly easier for carers to put the jacket on, as the child can be laid into the back section before fitting and fastening the front piece. The side-to-side design is particularly useful for severe scoliosis in older boys who have not had surgery when there are significant rotational elements and prominent rib protrusions. The child is laid supine to remove the deforming force of gravity during the casting process. Figure 10.10 shows a casting table/frame specifically designed for the purpose, although a similar effect can be achieved using foam blocks. Two key features are (1) the knee support to raise the legs and flex the knees, allowing and therefore mimicking an almost seated position whilst lying supine; and (2) a removable and adjustable bar located above the waist used to tie fabric around to support the patient around the waist area (Fig. 10.11). The band accentuates the waist in the cast which anchors the subsequent orthosis securely and limits

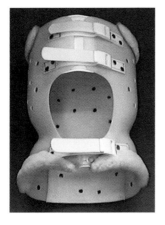

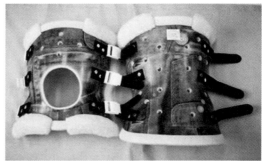

Fig. 10.7 One-piece wraparound TLSO.   **Fig. 10.8** Front and back bivalve TLSO.

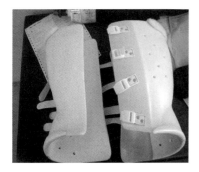

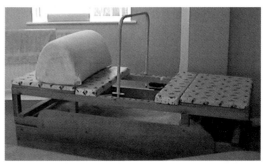

Fig. 10.9 Side-to-side bivalve TLSO.   **Fig. 10.10** A casting-couch for children with neuromuscular conditions.

migration of the orthosis under the arms. Padding is often helpful over the edges of the plastic under the arms and over the top of the thighs; the TLSO would be worn over a vest or T-shirt.

Becker muscular dystrophy

BMD is the relatively milder form of X-linked recessive muscular dystrophy and is caused by a partial deficiency of the protein dystrophin. The clinical appearance and distribution of muscle weakness is very similar to DMD but progression is much slower and contractures are therefore often less severe. It has a wide spectrum of severity; around 40% of patients lose the ability to walk independently although this occurs later than in boys with DMD, while others continue to walk for several decades (Dubowitz 1995). Cardiomyopathy is common and more likely to be symptomatic than in DMD (Quinlivan and Dubowitz 1992). The treatment principles described for boys with DMD apply to those with BMD and there may similarly be indications for using night AFOs and prolonging ambulation with KAFOs.

110

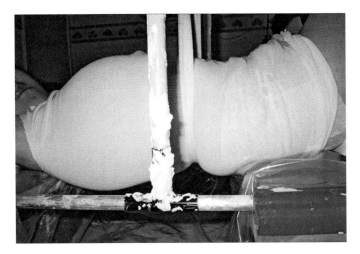

Fig. 10.11 Tying material around the child's midriff helps to accentuate the waist.

Spinal muscular atrophy

Spinal muscular atrophy (SMA) is an autosomal recessive disorder which manifests itself by degeneration of the anterior horn cells of the spinal cord, and in the most severe forms, of the bulbar motor nuclei, resulting in proximal and symmetrical muscle weakness. Children with SMA are often bright, with intelligence in the upper normal range despite their significant physical disability (von Gontard et al. 2002). Classification of SMAs is most usefully based on clinical severity (Munsat 1991) (Table 10.2).

SEVERE SMA (TYPE I/WERDNIG–HOFFMANN DISEASE)

Children with severe SMA present as floppy babies with progressive, severe, generalized weakness in the first few months of life. There is marked respiratory involvement and as a result they rarely survive beyond 2 years of age. Treatment will be mainly supportive. The orthotist may be involved in providing a supportive spinal jacket with a diaphragmatic aperture to help maintain a reclined sitting position without compromising respiratory function. Due to the small size of the infant and the severity of weakness, a softer rather than rigid material, is likely to be more appropriate.

TABLE 10.2
Classification of spinal muscular atrophy

Type	Onset	Course	Age at death
I (severe)	Birth to 6 months	Never sit	Usually < 2 years
II (intermediate)	< 18 months	Never stand	> 2 years
III (mild)	> 18 months	Stand alone	Adult

INTERMEDIATE SMA (TYPE II)

Weakness usually becomes apparent between 6 and 12 months of age and the child presents with inability to stand or walk. In contrast to severe SMA, children with intermediate and mild SMA can be expected to survive into adulthood, provided that respiratory function is not compromised and infections are either avoided or treated promptly. The limb joints are often hyperextendable, particularly at the elbow and hands, but are also prone to contractures related to immobility and positioning. However the weakness is generally non-progressive and standing and/or walking can be promoted with the use of a standing frame, custom-made thoracolumbar sacral hip–knee–ankle–foot orthosis (TLSH KAFO) (Fig. 10.12) or KAFOs depending on the child's proximal muscle strength (Granata et al. 1987); this intervention rarely needs to be combined with surgery to facilitate fitting.

The ankle is prone to develop equinus during growth and tend towards an over-pronated posture during standing. AFOs are often used as a preventative intervention to avoid fixed deformities either in the day or night-time; if the child is using a standing frame then AFOs may be helpful to promote a stable base. If KAFOs are provided then AFOs should be worn when KAFOs are not being used. Inclusion of a generous amount of padding is advisable inside the orthosis over the medial ankle, foot border and arch areas to avoid creating sores; Y-strapping can also be incorporated to supinate the ankle.

Smaller lighter children who require KAFOs to stand and walk can usually manage with an orthosis that only has a single lateral side member (omitting the medial hinge), resulting in a significant weight reduction. The structural integrity of the orthosis is maintained by extending the below-knee section of the orthosis to include the medial condyle of the knee and riveting this to the anterior knee section (Fig. 10.13). This design provides excellent control of knee valgus posture that is particularly common amongst SMA patients. The ability to walk in KAFOs may be maintained over many years, helping to

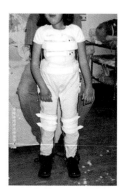

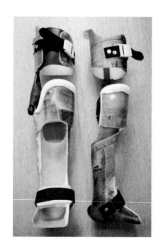

Fig. 10.12 Custom-made TLSHpKAFO to enable standing.

Fig. 10.13 John Florence lightweight KAFO for small children, such as those with SMA.

control both joint contractures and limit progressive scoliosis. Some children show functional improvement over time and, with appropriate training, may achieve progression from standing in a frame to walking with KAFOs. There has been some experimentation with providing reciprocating gait orthoses to children with SMA, but the outcomes are rather inconsistent.

Early and rapidly progressive scoliosis is commonly associated with Type II SMA and provision of a spinal orthosis early can reduce the rate at which the deformity progresses (Fig. 10.14). The child is cast for the TLSO in a supine position to remove the deforming force of gravity. A one-piece wraparound design is usually preferred and creating a window over the abdomen may relieve any feeling of restricted breathing, and is essential for children with gastrostomy. Drilling 8-10 mm diameter perforations in the back of the TLSO can decrease the weight and increase the flexibility of the orthosis; padding can be added where required or over the edges of the jacket rather than added as a lining throughout which can feel very hot for the child. The TLSO is always recommended to be worn over a T-shirt or vest. Spinal fusion may become necessary once the child is older providing they are otherwise fit enough from a respiratory perspective. If not, then designing an appropriate

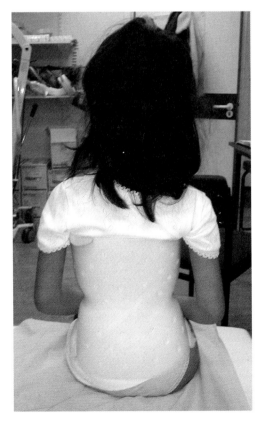

Fig. 10.14 TLSO for a child with SMA.

113

Fig. 10.15 CTLSO with flange to help support the head of a boy with SMA.

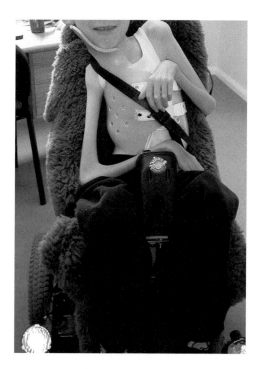

spinal orthosis to support the child's head can provide a challenge to the orthotist and seating specialists (Fig. 10.16). Spinal orthosis and spinal fusion are not usually compatible with continued mobility in KAFOs, since they limit compensatory trunk side flexion when the hip abductors are weak; however some children can disprove this presumption.

MILD SMA (TYPE III/KUGELBURG–WELANDER DISEASE)
The ability to walk is achieved at the normal age or slightly late and the child often presents with difficulty in the more advanced gross motor skills of hopping, running and jumping. Proximal weakness may give rise to a modified Gower's manoeuvre when getting up from the floor. The degree of muscle weakness is generally relatively static; and scoliosis and joint contractures are therefore rare in this group (Carter et al. 1995). Orthotic intervention, e.g. with foot orthoses or AFOs, may be helpful for children with ankle instability during standing and walking. However, any prolonged periods of immobility can result in the loss of walking ability altogether, and for these children rehabilitation can usually be achieved in KAFOs.

Congenital muscular dystrophy
The term congenital muscular dystrophy (CMD) describes a heterogeneous group of conditions presenting with muscle weakness at birth or early in infancy. These conditions are caused by autosomal recessive defects, and increasing use of more specific genetic tests means previously undifferentiated subgroups can now be distinguished on the basis of the

underlying molecular pathology and/or cerebral involvement. Achievement of the normal developmental motor milestones is usually delayed and some children may present with hypotonia while others have associated contractures or arthrogryposis at birth. With the exception of Fukuyama congenital muscular dystrophy, these conditions are generally static but there may be great variability in prognosis. Joint contractures may also develop insidiously and restrict function to a greater degree than muscle weakness if not controlled. There can be respiratory difficulties due to associated diaphragmatic involvement, in infancy or later in adolescence. The efficiency of nocturnal respiration can deteriorate and is a particular feature of the rigid spine phenotype which responds well to nocturnal nasal ventilation.

The child should be encouraged to be active, mobile and ambulant if possible from an early stage since immobility leads to further progression of contractures. It is particularly important to be vigilant and treat contractures promptly with regular passive stretching, serial casting and night-time orthoses. In some cases the child may need surgery to achieve standing or walking but this should be undertaken when the child displays some inclination to weight-bear; if undertaken prior to this time the deformities are likely to recur. In view of the heterogeneity of the condition it is difficult to make specific recommendations but spinal or lower-limb orthoses and standing-frames can be used judiciously to overcome activity limitations and limit deformity as necessary. The child's individual requirements can also change over time and it may be necessary to either increase or reduce orthotic support; therefore regular orthotic reviews are advisable.

Hereditary motor and sensory neuropathies (HMSN)
This group of disorders affects the peripheral sensory and motor nerves and forms of the condition have at times been labelled as Charcot–Marie–Tooth (CMT) disease and peroneal muscular atrophy (PMA) (Harding 1995). Most HMSN are dominantly inherited and the common forms are Type I (sub-forms are types 1a and 1b), a predominantly demyelinating form with delayed nerve-conduction times, and Type II which is a non-demyelinating axonal disorder in which nerve-conduction times preserved. Clinically the two forms are similar but type I generally appears at a younger age than type II.

Early signs are pes cavus (high arch) and an abnormal or clumsy gait. This clumsiness is partly due to distal muscle weakness, in particular dorsiflexor and peroneal muscles which predispose to inversion instability and intrinsic muscles causing retracted (hammer) toes, as well as sensory and proprioception impairment. The legs can take on a classical 'stork' leg appearance due to wasting of the lower legs. Increasing muscle imbalance around the ankles and feet exacerbates the equinus and cavovarus foot deformities and clawed toes along with the characteristic ataxic high stepping gait. Over time, without intervention, a once supple foot can become deformed and rigid with painful callosities under the metatarsal heads. Shoes can also become uncomfortable due to pressure and rubbing on the dorsum of the toes and stability during walking may become difficult if the hindfoot goes into significant varus. If sensory loss is severe, patients rely mainly on visual information to maintain balance and may also be prone to pressure sores or neuropathic ulcers.

When mild instability is present, insoles or foot orthoses may be the first line of treatment to correct or accommodate hindfoot varus and redistribute pressure under the foot. To assess how flexible is the hindfoot varus, place a small wedge under the lateral forefoot and see how much the hindfoot straightens. If the lateral forefoot wedge corrects the hindfoot then this can be incorporated into a foot orthosis (Figs 10.16, 10.17); and if not then the deformity must be accommodated. If there is a flaccid dropfoot (equinus in swing phase of gait only) then a posterior leaf-spring AFO can be provided to improve walking efficiency and reduce the risk of falling; a corrective Y-strap can be added to counter any varus tendency. Fixed AFOs will help to control progressive foot deformity more effectively than the leaf-spring design and provide greater stability; however significant reduced sensory awareness can make walking with a rigid AFO more difficult. Orthotic management should be combined with passive stretching of the muscle groups liable to shorten, predominantly gastrocnemius. Orthopaedic intervention will depend on the severity of the disease. When

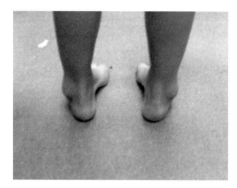
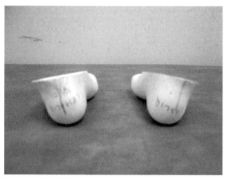

Fig. 10.16 Pes cavus and hindfoot varus associated with HMSN and the filled casts taken to produce foot orthoses; the medial arch area of the cast has been filled to permit midfoot pronation.

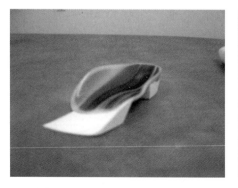
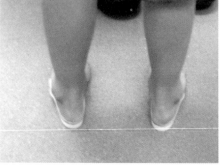

Fig. 10.17 Lateral wedging of the forefoot in the resulting foot orthosis helps to correct and control hindfoot varus; note the recess provided on the lateral border of the shell to accommodate the base of the 5th metatarsal.

equinus, cavus and varus deformities of the foot and ankle become severe, correction by osteotomy or arthrodesis may be necessary to relieve pain and preserve function but is usually considered in adulthood.

Whilst we have predominantly focused on the lower limbs, hand function is also compromised by weakness associated with HMSN interfering with writing and other necessary activities. A thumb-opposition orthosis may help to achieve a pinch grip and aid activities such as writing or eating. A wrist–hand orthosis, cast in a functional position and used at night, may help to prevent soft-tissue contracture when there is severe wasting of the thenar eminence.

Conclusions

Orthoses have a vital part to play in management of children with neuromuscular diseases. The range of biomechanical problems encountered is diverse and the possible orthotic solutions range from a simple insole or heel cup to a complex HKAFO or CTLSO. However, no matter what the objectives, or how good the methods and designs used to make the orthosis, failure will occur if the child is not wearing the orthosis consistently on a regular basis. Treatment outcomes are strongly influenced by the amount of time the orthosis is used and any non-compliance for even short periods of time can lead to poor results. Attempting to eliminate the reasons of non-compliances should be at the forefront in the decision to provide orthoses by using teamwork, careful assessment of the treatment objectives and identification of any biomechanical problem. Then the orthosis can be designed with a greater appreciation of the specific problems encountered in managing children with these conditions. In our experience, children with the conditions considered in this chapter have low pain thresholds and are often fragile. Although vacuum-forming is usually preferred for most applications so that orthoses are tight fitting, this is not generally the case for children these conditions; drape-forming over extra allowances results in a looser fit which increases compliance and aids the longevity of orthoses as children grow. There are a number of other neuromuscular conditions such as congenital myopathies and other dystrophies that can also be helped using the principles outlined in this chapter.

References

Bakker JPJ, De Groot IJM, Beckerman H, de Jong BA, Lankhorst GJ (2000) The effects of knee–ankle–foot orthoses in the treatment of Duchenne muscular dystrophy: review of the literature. *Clin Rehabil* **14**: 343–59.
Carter GT, Abresch RT, Fowler WM Jr, Johnson ER, Kilmer DD, McDonald CM (1995) Profiles of neuromuscular disease: spinal muscular atrophy. *Am J Phys Med Rehab* **74**: 150–9.
Dubowitz V (1995) *Muscle Disorders in Childhood, 2nd edn*. London: W.B. Saunders.
Eagle M, Baudouin SV, Chandler C, Giddings DR, Bullock R, Bushby K (2002) Survival in Duchenne muscular dystrophy: improvements in life expectancy since 1967 and the impact of home nocturnal ventilation. *Neuromusc Disord* **12**: 926–30.
Galasko CSB, Delaney C, Morris P. (1992) Spinal stabilisation in Duchenne Muscular Dystrophy. *J Bone Joint Surg Br* **74**: 210–214.
Gowers WR (1879) *Pseudohypertrophic Muscular Paralysis. A Clinical Lecture*. London: J. and A. Churchill.
Granata C, Cornelio F, Bonfiglioli S, Mattutini P, Merlini L (1987) Promotion of ambulation of patients with spinal muscular atrophy by early fitting of knee–ankle–foot orthoses. *Dev Med Child Neurol* **29**: 221–4.
Harding AE (1995) From the syndrome of Charcot, Marie and Tooth to disorders of peripheral myelin proteins. *Brain* **118**: 809–18.

Hyde SA, Scott OM, Goddard CM, Dubovitz V (1982) Prolongation of ambulation in Duchenne muscular dystrophy. *Physiotherapy* **68**: 105–8.

Hyde SA, Fløytrup I, Glent S, Kroksmark AK, Salling B, Steffensen BF, Werlauff U, Erlandsen M (2000) A randomised comparative study of two methods of controlling tendo achilles contracture in Duchenne muscular dystrophy. *Neuromusc Disord* **10**: 257–63.

Khodadadeh S, McClelland MR, Patrick JH, Edwards RH, Evans GA (1986) Knee moments in Duchenne muscular dystrophy. *Lancet* **6**: 544–55.

Manzur AY, Kuntzer T, Pike M, Swan A (2004) Glucocorticoid corticosteroids for Duchenne muscular dystrophy. *Cochrane Database Syst Rev* (2) CD003725.

Moxley RT 3rd, Ashwal S, Pandya S, Connolly A, Florence J, Mathews K, Baumbach L, McDonald C, Sussman M, Wade C (2005) Practice parameter: corticosteroid treatment of Duchenne dystrophy: report of the Quality Standards Subcommittee of the American Academy of Neurology and the Practice Committee of Child Neurology Society. *Neurology* **64**: 13–20.

Munsat TL (1991) Workshop report: International SMA collaboration. *Neuromusc Disord* **1**: 81.

Noble-Jamieson CM, Heckmatt JZ, Dubowitz V, Silverman M (1986) Effects of posture and spinal bracing on respiratory function in neuromuscular disease. *Arch Dis Child* **61**: 178–81.

Quinlivan RM, Dubowitz V (1992) Cardiac transplantation in Becker muscular dystrophy. *Neuomusc Disord* **2**, 165–7.

Rodillo EB, Fernandez-Bermejo E, Heckmatt JZ, Dubovitz V (1988) Prevention of rapidly progressive scoliosis in duchenne muscular dystrophy by prolonging walking with orthoses. *J Child Neurol* **3**: 269–74.

Scott OM, Hyde SA, Goddard C, Dubovitz V (1981) Prevention of deformity in Duchenne muscular dystrophy. *Physiotherapy* **67**: 177–180.

Seeger BR, Sutherland A, Clark MS (1990) Management of scoliosis in Duchenne muscular dystrophy. *Arch Phys Med Rehabil* **65**: 83–6.

Spencer GE Jr, Vignos PJ Jr (1962) Bracing for ambulation in childhood progressive muscular dystrophy. *J Bone Joint Surg* **44**: 234–42.

Sutherland DH, Olshen R, Cooper L, Wyatt M, Leach J, Mubarak S, Schultz P (1981) The pathomechanics of gait in Duchenne muscular dystrophy. *Dev Med Child Neurol* **23**: 3–22.

Thompson N, Quinlivan R (2004) Muscle disorders of childhood onset. In: Stokes M, Ashburn MA, eds. *Physical Management in Neurological Rehabilitation*. London: Elsevier Mosby. pp. 347–64.

Vignos PJ, Wagner MB, Karlinchak B, Katirji B (1996) Evaluation of a program for long-term treatment of Duchenne muscular dystrophy: experience at the University Hospitals of Cleveland. *J Bone Joint Surg Am* **78**: 1844–52.

von Gontard A, Backes M, Laufersweiler-Plass C, Wendland C, Lehmkuhl G, Zerres K, Rudnik-Schoneborn S (2002) Psychopathology and familial stress – comparison of boys with Fragile X syndrome and spinal muscular atrophy. *J Child Psychol Psychiat* **43**: 949–57.

11
MYELOMENINGOCOELE

Brigid Driscoll, Robert Novak and Luciano Dias

Myelomeningocoele is a developmental defect of the spinal cord and vertebral arches. There is failed closure of the posterior neuropore of the neural tube around 28 days of gestation. In addition there is failed fusion of the vertebral arches. As a result there is dysplasia of the spinal cord and its membranes. There is neurological deficit at and distal to the level of injury. It is most common in the lumbosacral region. There is a herniated sac through the dura and bone that rests beyond the surface plane of the back. The sac contains cerebrospinal fluid, arachnoid, pia, and abnormal neural elements. Closure of the sac should occur within the first 24 hours of delivery. This is a preventive measure against infection and further damage to the spinal cord. Due to the increased accuracy of in-utero detection, high-resolution ultrasound, maternal serum alpha fetoprotein test and amniocentesis, most infants with myelomeningocoele are delivered via C-section in order to prevent further damage to the spinal cord.

The prevalence of myelomeningocoele is 1/1000 live births. It is slightly more common in females than males, a 1.3:1 ratio. Myelomeningocoele has a combination of etiologies. There are environmental and genetic factors that contribute to neural tube defects (NTDs). The Center for Disease Control in the USA recommends that women take 400 μg of folic acid per day, which can reduce the risk of neural tube defects up to 70%. Other environmental factors that may contribute to NTDs are maternal insulin dependent diabetes and maternal use of anti-seizure medications. There is ongoing research to identify the genes that contribute to NTDs. Families that have a child born with myelomeningocoele have a 2%–5% increased chance of having a second child with an NTD, compared with a 0.1% chance in the general population.

There are many potential consequences of myelomeningocoele. There is a resultant paraparesis of the lower extremities and sensory deficits are also present. Bowel and bladder dysfunction can be present. It is important to note, however, that the sensory level of involvement is not always equal to the motor level. Congenital orthopedic deformities such as talipes equinovarus and hip dislocation are common findings. Hydrocephalus is present in 85%–90% of children with myelomeningocoele, according to McLone and Dias (2001). There is a restriction in the flow of cerebrospinal fluid, CSF, from its point of production to final absorption in the superior sagittal sinus. Rekate (2001) reported that at least 80% of infants with myelomeningocoele in the US receive a ventricular shunt. Due to the multiple and complex nature of the problems associated with this condition it is essential to treat patients who have myelomeningocoele with a team approach. The team includes the patient, caregivers, neurosurgeon, orthopaedic surgeon, urologist,

TABLE 11.1
Myelomeningocoele Manual Muscle Test

	LEFT	RIGHT	Comments (include range of motion limitations, spasticity, reflex movements, etc.)
Iliopsoas (L_1-2)			
Sartorius (L_1-3)			
Hip-adductors (L_2-4)			
Tensor fascia lata			
Gluteus medius (L_4-S_1)			
Gluteus maximus (L_5-S_1)			
Quadriceps (L_2-4)			
Medial hamstrings (L_4-S_2)			
Lateral hamstrings (L_4-S_1)			
Anterior tibialis (L_4-L_5)			
Posterior tibialis (L_4-L_5)			
Peroneus longus (L_5-S_1)			
Peroneus brevis (L_5-S_1)			
Gastrocnemius soleus (S_1-S_2)			
Extensor hallucis longus (S_1-S_2)			
Flexor hallucis longus (S_1-S_2)			
Extensor digitorum longus (L_4-S_1)			
Extensor digitorum brevis (L_4-S_1)			
Flexor digitorum longus (L_4-S_1)			
Flexor digitorum brevis (L_4-S_1)			
Lumbricals			

*Indicate increase ($\uparrow$) or decrease ($\downarrow$) in strength in comparison to previous test dated_____

Please note any significant information on other muscle groups unlisted above (i.e. EHB; Flex. HB; internal or external rotators)

X	=	X	=	X	=	Present	Unable to be graded, but working
10	=	5	=	N	=	Normal	Complete range of motion against gravity with full resistance
9	=	4	=	G	=	Good	Complete range of motion against gravity with moderate resistance
8	=	4–	=	G–	=	Good Minus	Complete range of motion against gravity with some resistance
7	=	3+	=	F+	=	Fair Plus	Complete range of motion against gravity with slight resistance
6	=	3	=	F	=	Fair	Complete range of motion against gravity
5	=	3–	=	F–	=	Fair Minus	Incomplete (greater than ½ way) range of motion, gravity eliminated, plus sight resistance
4	=	2+	=	P+	=	Poor Plus	Less than ½ way against gravity or full range of motion, gravity eliminated, plus slight resistance
3	=	2	=	P	=	Poor	Complete range of motion with gravity eliminated
2	=	2–	=	P–	=	Poor Minus	Incomplete range of motion with gravity eliminated
1	=	1	=	T	=	Trace	Contraction felt, no visible joint movement
0	=	0	=	0	=	Zero	No contraction felt in the muscle

orthotist, physical therapist, occupational therapist, social worker, psychologist, and nursing staff.

Myelomeningocoele is often categorized according to the level of injury to the spinal cord. The functional level of involvement can be determined by a manual muscle test (MMT) of the lower-extremity musculature (Table 11.1). The MMT is performed after delivery and before closure of the neural sac. There is a postoperative MMT 5–7 days post-closure. Additional MMTs are ideally performed at 3 months, 6 months, 12 months, 18 months, 24 months, and annually after the age of 2 years. The levels of involvement are categorized as thoracic–high-lumbar, low-lumbar, high-sacral, and low-sacral (Table 11.2). It is important to take into consideration that the functional level is not always consistent with the neurosurgical level when considering the potential of each individual child. Throughout the growth years, MMT is a particularly helpful tool for determining if a child has a tethered cord. A tethered cord occurs when there is traction on the spinal cord from scarring around the neonatal closure. It occurs primarily during the growth years, but can also happen during adulthood. Signs and symptoms include neurological deterioration, a decrease in muscle strength, changes in sensation, spasticity of the lower extremities, bowel and bladder changes, back or leg pain, and rapid progression of a scoliosis.

Early management

In addition to determining the level of involvement it is essential to determine any orthopaedic deformities present at birth. A thorough assessment of hip integrity, lower-extremity contractures and foot deformities is necessary. Limited lower-extremity muscle innervation results in the antagonist muscle group's inability to work against each other, which in turn results in orthopaedic deformities. Early management of deformities is crucial if the child is to attain typical developmental milestones, postural control and future standing/ambulation activities. Higher levels of spinal-cord involvement tend to increase the severity and prevalence of contractures. A total body splint is indicated to improve or prevent hip- and knee-flexion contractures, or control extreme positioning of hip abduction,

TABLE 11.2
Myelomeningocoele functional levels

Muscle group	Thoracic/ high lumbar	Low lumbar	High sacral	Low sacral
Hip-flexors	+/−	+	+	+
Hip-adductors	+/−	+	+	+
Hip-extensors	−	−	+	+
Hip-abductors	−	−	+	+
Knee-extensors	−	+	+	+
Knee-flexors	−	+medial/-lateral	+	+
Ankle-dorsiflexors	−	−	+/−	+
Ankle-plantarflexors	−	−	−	+/−

+ = MMT of 3 or greater muscle grade
− = MMT 2 or less of a muscle grade

flexion, and external rotation. It is important to take into account that hip flexion contractures at 30° and knee-flexion contractures at 20° are normal in unaffected infants.

Foot deformities also require early treatment. Flexible foot deformities due to limited muscle innervation such as equinovarus or calcaneovalgus can be treated with an ankle foot orthosis (AFO). This will prevent development of contractures and maintain a foot position for future plantigrade weight bearing activities. A rigid talipes equinovarus deformity can be treated with serial casting or splinting, however surgical intervention is necessary in the majority of cases. The surgical correction is performed around the age of 10 months. Orthotic management following surgical cast removal is a polypropylene AFO with a full-length footplate to maintain the corrected foot position. Timely physical therapy and orthotic management coordinated by the orthopaedic surgeon is necessary to provide the optimal potential for each individual child. Early education for positioning, handling, range of motion, and orthotic use is often indicated.

The purpose of orthotic intervention is to maintain alignment, prevent deformities, correct flexible deformities, and facilitate independent mobility/function. The orthosis can also protect the insensate limb. The importance of upright mobility and weight bearing are crucial for many reasons. Weight-bearing promotes bone growth and density, improved bowel and bladder function, respiratory benefits, psychosocial benefits, helps to limit the development of contractures, and enables other upright activities of daily living.

The materials utilized for orthotic intervention have changed over time, from the metal conventional systems to contemporary thermoplastic devices. Conventional metal and leather systems were heavy and difficult to fit. They provided inadequate stability of the foot and ankle in the transverse and coronal planes, adversely affecting the proximal joints. This also led to an increased incidence of pressure sores. The introduction of thermoplastics allowed total contact fitting. This improved overall alignment and function in the orthosis, along with decreasing the incidence of pressure sores. The thermoplastic devices are also lighter in weight and cosmetically more acceptable. It is important to note that orthotic devices and materials used for patients with myelomeningocoele need to be latex-free due to the high incidence of latex allergies.

Thoracic and high lumbar level

Children with thoracic and high lumbar level myelomeningocoele can have function of the hip-flexors and adductors, but quadriceps power is not usually present. Due to the high level of spinal-cord involvement, orthoses and assistive devices are essential for upright weight bearing and mobility. The devices need to control the trunk over the pelvis and lower limbs, and therefore need to cross and control the hip. Dias (2001) reported that patients with high-level lesions without innervation of the quadriceps are able to achieve some form of ambulation within the first 13 years of life. In a retrospective study at Children's Memorial Hospital, Chicago, out of 32 thoracic/high lumbar level patients only one was a 'community ambulator' as an adult. Factors that contribute to cessation of ambulation activities include development of hip- and knee-flexion contractures, a scoliosis that requires surgical intervention, and the generally high-energy cost required for upright mobility.

STANDING-FRAME

A standing-frame is the first orthotic device for weight-bearing activities (Fig. 11.1). This orthosis is introduced around 12 months of age, consistent with normal development for standing activities. The standing-frame has a wide platform base with footplates allowing control of foot position and lower-extremity rotation. There is a circumferential knee component that controls the sagittal and coronal planes in order to promote knee extension with the lower extremities a shoulder width apart. There is a posterior gluteal pad to promote hip extension. The standing frame should also have a flexible thoracic corset for sagittal and coronal control of the trunk. Use of solid AFOs in conjunction with the standing-frame ensures weight-bearing with a plantigrade foot position, and maintains the foot in a subtalar neutral position. This is important to prevent varus or valgus deformities of the ankle and foot. The standing-frame assists in developing postural control, trunk strength, balance and righting reactions, and formation of the hip joints. Children are also able to better use their upper extremities and develop fine-motor skills. Around 18 months of age, or when the child expresses interest, an orthotic device that promotes independent mobility can be introduced.

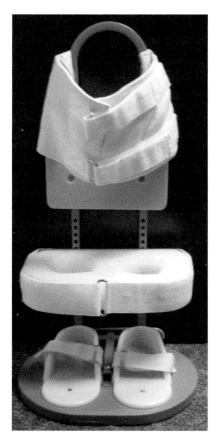

Fig. 11.1 Standing-frame.

PARAPODIUM

The parapodium is often selected when the patient has poor sitting balance, spasticity of the upper extremities or increased spinal deformities. The device is introduced around the age of two years and can be utilized as a standing-frame and as a form of mobility. Forward movement is initiated with upper-trunk and upper-extremity rotation. This device can also be used with a walker or forearm crutches using a swing-through gait pattern. The original parapodium was designed at the Ontario Crippled Children's Centre, Toronto, and has an oval platform base with tubular sidebars. There is a thoracic support piece along with an anterior knee bar. Hip and knee hinges can be unlocked to allow for sitting or locked in extension for upright posture. An additional anterior extension assist bar was a later addition to the platform, allowing the patient to pull-to-stand. The Rochester Parapodium is a similar device (Fig. 11.2). The hip and knee hinges are attached with flat sidebars and act independently in order to allow a more gradual descent into sitting from standing. The joints need only one hand to release them, allowing more balance and support from the free limb.

The ORLAU swivel-walker is also available. This device does not have hip or knee joints and therefore cannot be used for sitting. Two footplates are attached to the heavy platform base and are mounted so that only one can be flat on the floor at any time at which point the other plate is unloaded. Provided the centre of gravity is forward of the bearing centre, when the child leans or rotates their head, arms and trunk so that only one footplate is on the supporting surface, the base plate rotates forward on the unsupported side. Using this method only minimal coordination is required to facilitate locomotion and no walking aid is required.

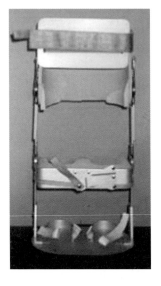

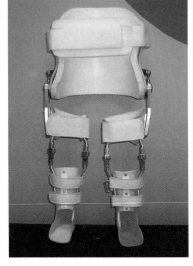

Fig. 11.2 Rochester parapodium.   **Fig. 11.3** Reciprocating gait orthosis (RGO).

RECIPROCATING GAIT ORTHOSIS

The reciprocating gait orthosis (RGO) (Fig. 11.3) may be considered when the child has hands-free sitting balance and minimal spinal deformities. The RGO is used with a walking aid, most often a reverse walker, and some children with increased postural control and trunk strength are able to progress towards ambulation with Canadian crutches. The system consists of a thoracic and pelvic section with posteriorly mounted cables attached to both hip hinges and bilateral KAFOs. Locking the hip hinge restricts the range of hip flexion and extension to what is useful during gait. A thigh cuff for the KAFO is necessary if knee-flexion contractures up to 20° are present, in order to promote knee extension or if there is a need to control knee position in the coronal plane. Forward propulsion is initiated by a lateral weight shift to unload the swing limb, and trunk extension to advance the swing limb forward with simultaneous extension of the stance limb.

The RGO was later designed with a single horizontal cable to eliminate the bulkiness of the double cable system. It is a lighter device that performs essentially in the same fashion. The isocentric RGO replaced all posterior cables on the system with a centrally pivoting posterior bar on the thoracic piece that attaches to bilateral hip joints. It is a significantly heavier device than the previously described RGOs but creates less friction. A hip hinge that additionally allows movement in the coronal plane when not weight-bearing may make self-catheterization easier. Phillips et al. (1995) and Guidera et al. (1993) have stated that an RGO can be fit for children with hip flexion contractures up to 35° and 45° respectively. However, hip-flexion contractures ranging from 30°–40° will result in a significantly shortened stride length. Katz et al. (1997) reported that use of the isocentric RGO provides a faster, more energy-efficient gait than the locked hip–knee–ankle–foot orthosis (HKAFO) in thoracic-level patients with myelomeningocoele.

HIP-GUIDANCE ORTHOSIS

The parawalker or hip guidance orthosis (HGO) was developed at the Orthotic Research and Locomotor Assessment Unit in Oswestry, UK. The orthosis maintains abduction of the hips using rigid hip hinge sections attached to conventional knee–ankle–foot orthoses (KAFOs) and heavy footplates. The hip hinge allows limited flexion and extension in a friction-free system for walking, and can be unlocked for sitting. Ambulation with this device is achieved using either crutches or a walker. Lateral weight shift of the trunk is combined with downward force through the assistive mobility device to extend the stance hip. Consequently the unloaded swing limb advances forward allowing a reciprocal walking pattern. This device can be used on a variety of surfaces including grass and inclines.

HIP–KNEE–ANKLE–FOOT ORTHOSIS

As well as the modular HKAFO systems, there may be occasions when a contemporary design of HKAFO is more appropriate. This device has a pelvic band which connects to single or double sidebars with thigh cuffs and an AFO section. There are separate hip and knee joints. Single or double sidebars are determined based on patient size and level of activity. The sidebars are most often made of aluminium, but can also be made of steel or titanium. Based on the level of involvement and abdominal strength it is essential to properly

125

choose a pelvic band. In order to increase the lever arm for more trunk and pelvic support, the pelvic band needs to be wider to increase the surface area. This prevents excessive forward flexion of the thorax and hips, and does not promote an increase in lumbar lordosis. Therefore a pelvic band with superior and inferior extensions, a butterfly band, may be indicated over a standard pelvic band for improved end-point control. The HKAFO controls lower-extremity rotation, joint motion in the sagittal plane at the hip, knee and ankle, and limits lateral leaning of the trunk due to weak hip-abductors. Modifications can be made to control excessive motion at the knee in the coronal plane. This could include varus or valgus leather straps or thermoplastic extensions on the AFO or thigh cuff. The hip and knee joints should have drop locks. The drop locks at the hip can be free or engaged during ambulation based on muscle strength and joint stability. The child needs active hip-flexors to use this device. Children can use a 4-point or swing-through gait pattern in order to achieve forward mobility. A walker, Canadian crutches or quad canes can be used for an assistive device.

Low-lumbar level

Children with low lumbar level lesions usually have active hip-flexors, hip-adductors, knee-extensors, and knee-flexors, especially medial hamstrings. Hip-extensors and abductors, and ankle-plantarflexors and dorsiflexors are absent. Due to the number of active muscles it is no longer necessary for an orthosis to cross the hip joint. These children more often than not still require the use of an assistive device. Occasionally children who do not have a shunt are able to walk without an assistive device. The retrospective study at Children's Memorial Hospital, Chicago, stated that 79% of low-lumbar level patients with myelomeningocoele remain 'community ambulators' into their adult years. There are some typical gait findings within this level of involvement because of the weak ankle plantarflexors and the gluteus muscles. Vankoski et al (1995) reported that there was a significant increase in anterior pelvic tilt, hip flexion, pelvic obliquity, and decreased walking velocity 60% slower than normal walking. A lateral trunk lean is noted on the stance leg due to weakness of the gluteus medius to control the coronal plane, reducing the external hip adduction moment, and to allow hip flexion of the opposite lower extremity for swing. A decrease in step length is noted due to the lack of antagonist hip muscles for pelvic stabilization. There is also increased hip and knee flexion in stance from ankle plantarflexor weakness. Moore et al. (2001) reported that individuals with low lumbar level myelomeningocoele can have a more efficient gait using a swing-through gait compared to a reciprocal gait pattern, walking faster using less energy; therefore many of them will prefer this technique.

KNEE–ANKLE–FOOT ORTHOSIS

The KAFO may be indicated for patients with low-lumbar involvement (Fig. 11.4). The KAFO consists of a total contact thermoplastic thigh cuff and AFO sections. Medial and lateral aluminum sidebars and a knee joint attach the two pieces. The thermoplastic components better distribute pressure and increase triplanar correction of the extremity. Depending on the desired planar motion control, there are a variety of orthotic knee hinges to choose from. Knee hinges are usually single axis and can be used with or without drop

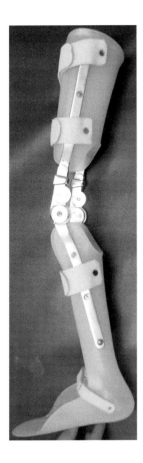

Fig. 11.4 Knee–ankle–foot orthosis (KAFO) with a dial lock distal to the mechanical joint for range of motion adjustability.

locks. If the quadriceps has a functional strength of at least 3+/5, then the sagittal plane can remain unrestricted. The sliding drop lock or ring lock uniformly covers the hinge proximal to the mechanical axis of the joint center. The drop lock can be held proximally off the hinge with a ball-bearing retainer to allow for free motion of the mechanical and anatomical joints. A variety of orthotic knee hinges can be used with this population. Step-locks allow for a ratcheting mechanism to lock in various sagittal knee positions as the joint is extended. Dial locks are used with soft-tissue flexion contractures; this allows easy adjustability with changes in range of motion. Future development of stance control knee joints for the pediatric population holds promise for improved motion during swing and stability during stance as well as a reduction in the weight of orthoses that cross the knee.

The indication for the KAFO may be for greater control of knee varus or valgus deformities. To better control these coronal deformities the thigh cuff or AFO sections may be extended along the knee to control excessive movement into varus or valgus. There is also the option of leather varus or valgus control knee straps. Finally, if a patient presented with rotary instability the use of a thermoset or laminate system will increase the durability of the device and better control the transverse plane.

TWISTER CABLES

Bilateral solid AFOs attached to a pelvic band with 'twister' cables (Fig. 11.5) may be used to control rotational deformities of the lower extremities. The twister system includes a leather covered aluminium pelvic band and flexible torque cables on the lateral aspect of the thigh that counteract medial or lateral rotational forces. The device can be assembled to externally or internally rotate the hip as needed in order to improve the child's foot-progression angle. The motion of hip and knee hinges is unrestricted in the sagittal plane and these components attach to bilateral solid AFOs. External tibial torsion is common in children with myelomeningocoele. Children with talipes equinovarus deformities or L4 lesion levels, due to unopposed medial hamstrings, tend to present with an associated internal tibial torsion. Twister orthoses may be cumbersome, but neglecting rotational deformities can have a detrimental effect on the child's balance and gait. If rotational deformities do not correct by the age of 5 or 6 years, a tibial derotation osteotomy may be indicated. The twister cables can also provide proprioceptive sensory input for stabilization of the lower extremities.

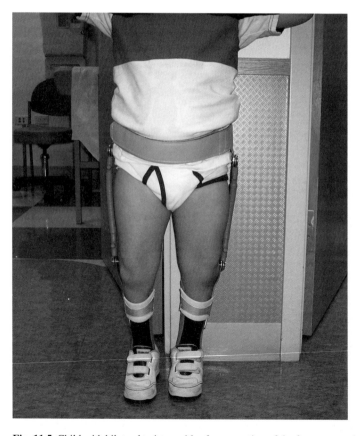

Fig. 11.5 Child with bilateral twister cables for correction of the foot progression angle.

GROUND REACTION ANKLE–FOOT ORTHOSIS

The Saltiel 'floor reaction ankle–foot orthosis' or 'ground reaction AFO' is a useful option for the patient with myelomeningocoele who exhibits proper mechanical alignment of the lower extremity, but demonstrates excessive knee flexion during stance (Fig. 11.6) The ground reaction AFO is able to create a knee-extension moment, providing (1) it has an adequate proximal, anterior lever arm, (2) it prevents dorsiflexion to limit anterior translation of the tibia during stance phase, and (3) it has a stiff full-length footplate to advance of the centre of pressure distally on the foot during stance phase. The child can be considered a candidate for a ground reaction AFO if the knee joint has soft-tissue flexion contractures of 5° or less; however, full range of extension is ideal. An important technique when casting for a ground reaction AFO is to maintain the ankle in 3°–5° of plantarflexion. This will facilitate the 'plantarflexion/knee-extension couple' by allowing the ground reaction force to proceed anterior to the knee-joint centre during stance phase. It is also important to assess and incorporate the appropriate thigh–foot angle during an impression as the lever arm of the footplate is compromised when there is a significant internal or external foot progression.

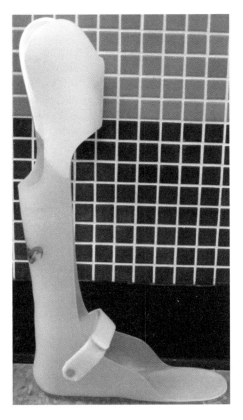

Fig. 11.6 Ground reaction ankle–foot orthosis (GRAFO) with reinforcing carbon fiber inserts to increase the mechanical stability of the orthosis.

This topic will be discussed further in the AFO section. Frequently carbon fibre reinforcements are applied at the ankle during vacuum-forming of the thermoplastic to make the orthosis more rigid and prevent failure into dorsiflexion. This fabrication technique is most important when a patient's weight or activity level is affecting durability of the orthosis. It is important to realise, when introducing the anterior ground reaction AFO to a child, that an adjustment period may be needed. Children need to develop increased proximal strength and postural control to counter the hip flexion created by the anterior ground reaction force. Consequently their gait can appear unsteady and inefficient when the device is initially introduced.

ANKLE–FOOT ORTHOSIS

The solid AFO is the most commonly used orthotic device for children with myelomeningocoele (Fig. 11.7). The AFO controls the foot and ankle. An AFO provides support for ankle plantarflexion and dorsiflexion activity, thus allowing foot clearance during gait, and avoiding excessive advancement of the tibia over the foot during stance. Indication for an AFO is a quadriceps muscle test grade of 3/5 or greater, and hamstrings of 2+/5. If hamstrings are not present children cannot use a conventional AFO due to the inability to

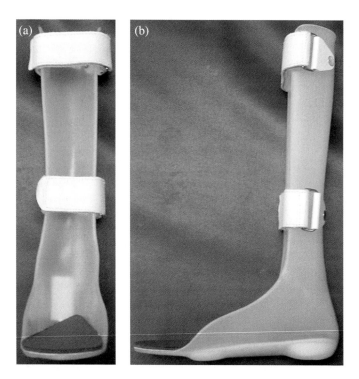

Fig. 11.7 (a) Coronal view of solid AFO with internal foot orthosis (FO). The FO has medial hindfoot and medial forefoot posts to provide an external supination moment. (b) Sagittal view of a solid AFO and internal FO with medial hindfoot and forefoot posts.

control the pelvis. When fabricating this orthosis it is essential to correct any flexible foot deformities within the impression. Ideally the ankle should be set in 0° of dorsiflexion to avoid knee flexion in stance and with the subtalar joint in neutral. Children can develop varus or valgus deformities due to muscle imbalance at the ankle and foot. It is essential to mould and fit an AFO properly, with correction of the above-mentioned flexible deformities, in order to prevent progression towards fixed deformity. Polypropylene is most commonly used when fabricating an AFO. It is very important to consider the rigidity of the plastic and geometry (i.e. corrugation or radius) of the orthosis, based on the patient's age, weight and activity level, in order to adequately control ankle dorsiflexion, crouch gait and closed-chain pronation. Copolymer should only be used with children who are very young and light. Assessment of plastic stress at the ankle should be performed during fitting to ensure the orthosis is adequately constructed. Trim-lines anterior to the malleoli can increase control in the sagittal and coronal plane at the ankle and foot. The deep trim-line will increase durability at the ankle to prevent sagittal stress or fractures in the plastic. In addition, pad placement along the tibia can increase varus or valgus control at the subtalar joint. A full-length footplate provides the option of extending the sidewalls of the orthosis in order to control excessive forefoot abduction or adduction. The full-length footplate is indicated for toe-clawing which is often present in this population, and allows the option of using a metatarsal pad to offload the metatarsal heads. The increased length will also provide a longer lever arm in order to produce a knee-extension moment, and keep the centre of mass posterior. Finally the full-length footplate allows longer use of the AFO based on more growth potential. It is important to consider the width of the straps based on the size of the child, and how much force is being transferred into the strap. A wide strap, or the use of proximal and distal calf straps, can reduce pressure on the anterior aspect of the tibia, thus preventing development of skin irritation or ulcers.

An important clinical assessment when determining the effectiveness of a solid AFO is the thigh–foot angle (TFA) (Fig. 11.8). This measurement of tibial torsion, as described by Staheli (1997), is performed by placing the ankle in subtalar neutral and determining the angle between the longitudinal axis of the femur and the longitudinal axis of the foot through the third toe, using a goniometer. Vankoski et al. (2000) demonstrated that in patients with lumbosacral myelomeningocoele and tibial torsion >20°, the effectiveness of the solid AFO was compromised. The limitation of the AFO was evident at mid-stance when the magnitude of the knee-extension moment was reduced. Presence of 30° external tibial torsion may lead to 25% reduction in the knee-axis lever-arm length. Therefore it is necessary to evaluate a patient's TFA in order to assess the potential effectiveness of a solid AFO.

High sacral level
Children with high sacral-level lesions have active hip-flexors, extensors, abductors, adductors, knee-flexors and extensors. Ankle dorsiflexors may or may not be present and ankle plantarflexors are absent. Findings at Children's Memorial Hospital, Chicago, show that 94% of individuals with sacral-level myelomeningocoele remain 'community ambulators' as adults. These children typically ambulate with solid AFOs without needing assistive mobility devices. Their gait pattern may display an increased anterior pelvic tilt

Fig. 11.8 Staheli method of tibial torsion measurement.

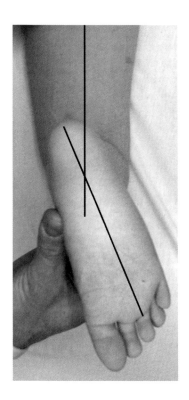

and pelvic obliquity due to weakness in the gluteus maximus and medius. A hinged AFO is not indicated for children with this level of involvement due to weak ankle plantarflexors. A hinged AFO would allow excessive advancement of the tibia over the foot leading to a crouch gait. This places stress on the knee joints and lead to the development of hip and knee flexion contractures.

Low sacral level
Children with low sacral-level involvement have complete innervation of hip and knee muscles. Ankle dorsiflexors and plantarflexors are also present, but they may be weak. These children do not require any mobility aids for ambulation. There is a normal anterior pelvic tilt and little increase in range of pelvic obliquity as the hip muscles provide stability in stance. Similarly, increased lateral trunk motion associated with weak hip muscles is not seen in children with low sacral lesions. Choosing the appropriate orthotic device for this particular child can be difficult and should be closely monitored. Close assessment of strength and endurance is necessary. If the plantarflexor strength is less than 3/5 the child will probably still require the use of a solid AFO. Use of a thinner polypropylene or even copolymer may be possible as long as it does not allow a crouch gait. A hinged AFO with a plantarflexion stop and free dorsiflexion can be an additional orthotic option, however a posterior dorsiflexion control strap can be added to the orthosis in order to limit excessive translation of the tibia over the foot.

SUPRAMALLEOLAR ORTHOSIS

Use of a supramalleolar orthosis (SMO) may be indicated when the plantarflexor strength and endurance are enough to prevent a crouch gait but a tendency for ankle instability persists (Fig. 11.9). The circumferential SMO controls the hindfoot, midfoot, and forefoot. Proper moulding in subtalar neutral during the impression ensures an optimal fit, and overall improved alignment of the foot in the SMO. The slightly increased lever arm from the malleolar extensions provide medial and lateral control if excessive hindfoot varus or valgus are present. Extrinsic hindfoot and forefoot posting, with plastic, ethylene vinyl acetate (EVA) or dense crepe, can be used for additional varus and valgus control.

FOOT ORTHOSIS

If control of foot posture is all that is required, the child can use a semi-rigid foot orthosis. Due to the sensory deficits that are often present in this population, a rigid thermoplastic foot orthosis should probably be avoided to prevent the risk of ulcers. The semi-rigid or multi-durometer insert lasts about 6 months to a year depending on the size and activity level of the child. The integrity of the foot orthosis needs to be monitored closely to ensure proper positioning and padding of the foot to prevent ulceration. Semi-rigid orthoses are made of materials such as EVA and polyurethane foams. Dense crepe or cork can be added to the base of the orthosis to influence foot alignment. Medial posting of the orthosis aims to control pronatory forces; lateral posting aims to counter supinatory forces.

Scoliosis/kyphosis

Locke et al. (2001) stated that scoliosis develops in approximately 60% of children with myelomeningocoele. Of these, according to Müller and Nordwall (1992), 94% are thoracic-level while only 20% are sacral-level. Paralytic scoliosis is most common but congenital scoliosis also occurs.

THORACOLUMBAR–SACRAL ORTHOSIS (TLSO)

The purpose of a TLSO is to decrease the rate of curve progression, and avoid or delay the need for spinal fusion until skeletal maturity. An additional goal of the TLSO is to restore

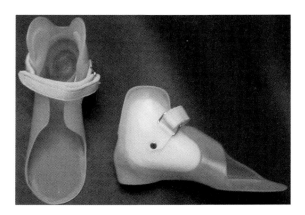

Fig. 11.9 Bilateral supramalleolar orthoses (SMO). The full-length footplate and extended lateral trim-line limit pronation and excessive forefoot abduction.

133

the follower load of the spinal column by ensuring the head is positioned over the pelvis in the coronal plane (Patwardhan et al. 1999). The TLSO can be used with flexible paralytic curves greater than 30°, or with congenital curves that have superior or inferior flexible segments. Scoliosis management with the TLSO is for daytime use while the child is upright.

The most commonly used TLSO is the anterior opening TLSO made of polyethylene (Fig. 11.10). This orthotic style allows for more growth and adjustability. A bivalve TLSO is an alternative design, but the seam where the anterior and posterior sections join can prove to be a problem with growth. Children with higher levels of involvement can also use a flexible foam TLSO (Fig. 11.11). The orthosis is made of dense foamed EVA that is reinforced with a thermoplastic exoskeleton for durability. This orthosis does not provide as much curve correction, but is better tolerated with children who have poor trunk control and in respect to skin integrity. Pelvic obliquity is quite common in children with myelomeningocoele and is a contributing factor to paralytic curves. It is therefore essential to capture the pelvis and correct any pelvic obliquity while taking an impression for a TLSO. Once the orthosis is provided it may be necessary to assess the child's seating system to minimize pelvic obliquity, and to maintain the trunk over the pelvis. It is also important to assess any changes in functional ability when the child is wearing a TLSO. The TLSO may make standing or walking, and other functional activities more difficult, this should be systematically assessed. Further modifications may be necessary, and in some cases a TLSO may no longer be considered beneficial if it adversely affects function beyond a reasonable capacity.

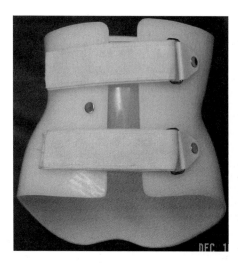 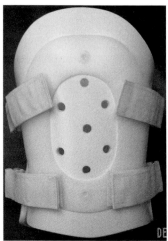

Fig. 11.10 Thoracolumbar–sacral orthosis (TLSO) with an anterior opening.

Fig. 11.11 Bivalve soft foam TLSO with more rigid polyethylene exoskeleton.

Night orthotic management

There is often an indication for orthotic management at night for children with myelo-meningocoele. As we have described this is especially important with infants. Management of contractures is essential to allow optimal function. Night orthotic management can improve range of motion limitations, prevent surgery, or at least lengthen tissues in order to prepare a child for surgery. Night-time AFO splinting may be indicated for infants with foot deformities (Fig. 11.12), and the requirement may persist throughout childhood. This can be for equinovarus foot deformities, complications from a tethered cord, or previous poor management. Children may require the use of an AFO to improve alignment for a weight-bearing orthosis or prevent surgery. The AFO splints are often made from polyethylene in order to increase comfort and therefore compliance for night use. An anterior shell or multiple-strap system can be used to keep the AFO and foot in appropriate alignment. Low-temperature plastics moulded directly to the child may also be used. If the child is very young and growing quickly a low-temperature plastic is often more economical and time efficient. This is also true with the older child who may have several devices made in a program of serial splinting.

Knee contractures may be treated with a night KAFO made of polyethylene or copolymer. The use of 'dial' or 'step' incremental locking knee hinges for knee contractures enables easy modification in order to accommodate changes in joint range of motion. It is

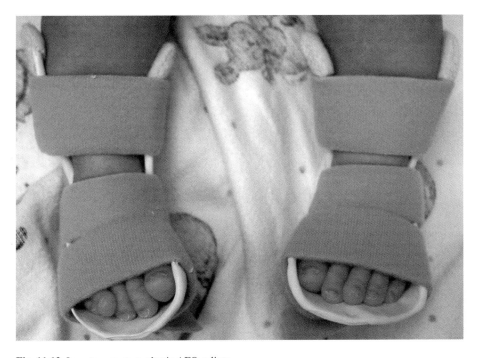

Fig. 11.12 Low-temperature plastic AFO splints.

Fig. 11.13 Low-temperature plastic anterior total body splint (TBS). Child is also wearing bilateral low-temperature AFOs.

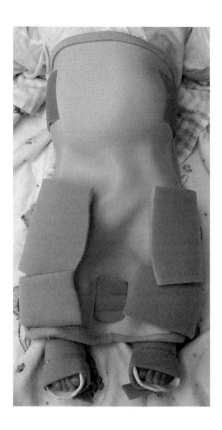

necessary to provide appropriate strapping to ensure the correct alignment is maintained between the orthosis and the limb. Another option is a total-contact bivalve design to increase the range of knee motion.

Children with higher levels of impairment and who require control of the trunk, pelvis, and lower extremities can benefit from the use of a total body splint (TBS) (Fig. 11.13). The anterior TBS is generally made from low-temperature plastic moulded directly to the child. The posterior TBS can alternatively be made from high-temperature plastic. It is a posterior lumbar sacral orthosis (LSO) attached to bilateral KAFOs without knee hinges. Rotation in the lower extremities can be controlled in the transverse plane if the distal sections include the foot. Aluminum bars are used to provide a substructure across the trunk and leg components, and provide ease for growth adjustments. A simple foam wedge can also be used to control hip abduction or adduction.

Education, and care of orthoses
It is crucial to educate the child, family, caregivers and other health-care professionals on the appropriate use and maintenance of any orthosis. Improper use of an orthotic device can decrease function, have negative effects on alignment, and create serious skin problems. Proper instruction for donning and doffing needs to be provided verbally during the

fitting, and supplemented with written instructions whenever necessary. It is often helpful to have the child and caregiver demonstrate these tasks during the fitting appointment to ensure the instructions are understood. Due to the sensory deficits present in children with myelomeningocoele it is important to educate the child and family about proper skin care. Examination of skin integrity, especially along the soles of the feet, should become a daily routine in order to prevent the development of skin ulcers. If any irritation is noted the child and caregivers should be instructed to contact the orthotist immediately for orthotic adjustments in order to prevent skin breakdown. Daily cleansing of the skin is also important to prevent skin irritation, athlete's foot or rashes that can be exacerbated by using plastic orthoses. Plastic orthoses should be cleaned regularly with mild soap and water or alcohol to avoid any skin irritation. A pressure sore or ulcer needs immediate treatment upon identification. When these factors are taken into consideration, together with the technical issues, the overall orthotic treatment plan will be much more successful.

Summary

Although the exact causes remain unknown, advances in antenatal detection and improving maternal nutrition are reducing the prevalence of myelomeningocoele. When a child does have a myelomeningocoele the resulting paralysis and neuromuscular function should be monitored using regular manual muscle tests. Determination of active muscle groups, their strength and level of function will assist the team in providing the most appropriate physical management program and orthotic intervention. Children with thoracic and high-lumbar level lesions may use a parapodium, swivel walker, hip guidance orthosis, reciprocating gait orthosis, or a contemporary HKAFO. However it is likely that children with thoracic and high-lumbar lesions will use a wheelchair as their main form of mobility as adults. When the level of the lesion is determined to be low-lumbar, the team may choose from KAFOs, twister cables attached to AFOs, ground reaction AFOs, or solid AFOs. A child with a high-sacral level lesion often ambulates with a solid ankle–footorthosis and without mobility aids. Children with low sacral-level lesions may use AFOs or foot orthoses. Whatever the level of lesion, the emphasis must be for a team approach to educate the child, family and caregivers in the appropriate use of orthoses as a vital component of the comprehensive care of children with myelomeningocoele.

References

Dias LS (2001) Expected long-term walking ability. In: Sarwark JF, Lubicky JP, eds. *Caring for the Child with Spina Bifida*. Chicago, IL: American Academy of Orthopaedic Surgery, pp. 261–2.

Guidera KJ, Smith S, Raney E, Frost J, Pugh L, Griner D, Ogden JA (1993) Use of the reciprocating gait orthosis in myelodysplasia. *J Pediatr Orthop* **13**: 341–8.

Katz DE, Haideri N, Song K, Wyrick P (1997) Comparative study of conventional hip-knee-ankle-foot orthoses versus reciprocating-gait orthoses for children with high-level paraparesis. *J Pediatr Orthop* **17**: 377–86.

Locke MD, Dias LS, Sarwark JF (2001) The relationship between infrapelvic obliquity and scoliosis. In: Sarwark JF, Lubicky JP, eds. *Caring for the Child with Spina Bifida*. Chicago, IL: American Academy of Orthopaedic Surgery, pp. 105–15.

McLone DG, Dias MS (2001) Hydrocephalus and the Chiari II malformation in myelomeningocele. In: Sarwark JF, Lubicky JP, eds. *Caring for the Child with Spina Bifida*. Chicago, IL: American Academy of Orthopaedic Surgery, pp. 29–42.

Moore CA, Nejad B, Novak RA, Dias LS (2001) Energy cost of walking in low lumbar myelomeningocele. *J Pediatr Orthop* **21**: 388–91.

Müller EB, Nordwall A (1992) Prevalence of scoliosis in children with myelomeningocele in western Sweden. *Spine* **9**: 1097–102.

Patwardhan AG, Havey RM, Meade KP, Lee B, Dunlap B (1999) A follower load increases the load-carrying capacity of the lumbar spine in compression. *Spine* **24**: 1003–9.

Phillips DL, Field RE, Broughton NS, Menelaus MB (1995) Reciprocating orthoses for children with myelomeningocele: a comparison of two types. *J Bone Joint Surg Br* **77B**: 110–13.

Rekate HL (2001) Pathophysiology and management of hydrocephalus in spina bifida. In: Sarwark JF, Lubicky JP, eds. *Caring for the Child with Spina Bifida*. Chicago, IL: American Academy of Orthopaedic Surgery, pp. 395–407.

Staheli LT (1997) Torsional deformities. *Pediatr Clin North Am* **24**: 799.

Vankoski SJ, Sarwark JF, Moore C, Dias L (1995) Characteristic pelvic, hip, and knee kinematic patterns in children with lumbosacral myelomeningocele. *Gait Posture* **3**: 51–7.

Vankoski SJ, Michaud S, Dias L (2000) External tibial torsion and the effectiveness of the solid ankle–foot orthoses. *J Pediatr Orthop* **20**: 349–55.

12
IDIOPATHIC SCOLIOSIS

Paul Horwood

Scoliosis is defined as any structural curvature of the spine in the coronal plane of greater than 10° as measured by the Cobb method (Cobb 1948). Scoliosis is often associated with rotational deformity in the transverse plane or with kyphosis, which is excessive forward curvature of the spine in the sagittal plane. The term idiopathic scoliosis is used when there is no known aetiology and is therefore a diagnosis of exclusion – hence the importance of undertaking a full family and medical history and a thorough physical examination (Burgoyne and Fairbank 2001). The aetiology of idiopathic scoliosis (IS) is unknown but it is believed to be multifactorial (Lowe et al. 2000). Scoliosis is also associated with many neuromuscular conditions such as muscular dystrophy, myelomeningocoele and cerebral palsy due to muscle strength imbalance and weakness. However, this chapter focuses predominantly on the orthotic management of idiopathic scoliosis in which the child usually has the ability to partially correct his or her own posture.

IS can be classified by age of onset, using the terms 'infantile' (IIS), with onset below the age of 3 years; 'juvenile' (JIS), with onset between 3 and 10 years; and 'adolescent' (AIS), from 11 years to maturity. However, this corresponds to age at diagnosis and may not be consistent with the actual age at curve development (Bradford et al. 1987). In the early-onset types of scoliosis, IIS and JIS, about 20% of patients may not truly have an idiopathic aetiology, in that they may have neuro-axis anomalies that contribute to curve development (Dobbs et al. 2001). In an unpublished audit of the diagnoses of children provided with spinal orthoses at the Nuffield Orthopaedic Centre in Oxford, UK, we found that most were found to have some identifiable pathology, and so their scoliosis was not, by definition, idiopathic.

Scoliosis curves are further defined as being either primary or secondary, with the primary curve being the more rigid and severe deformity. The secondary curve is considered to be compensatory to the primary problem and is usually flexible, although it can become more rigid over time (Moe et al. 1978). The secondary curve develops in an attempt to maintain the head positioned over the pelvis (Burgoyne and Fairbank 2001). Curves are described as left or right depending on direction of the convexity, with the apex being at the vertebrae most displaced from the sagittal-plane midline. Spinal curvatures themselves may be further classified by their vertebral apex position (Table 12.1). The most common curve patterns (in descending frequency) are right thoracic double curves consisting of right thoracic and left lumbar, thoracolumbar and lumbar curves.

The prevalence of scoliosis greater than 10° is reported to be around 2%–4% of the population (Cassella and Hall 1991). Epidemiological studies based on school screening

TABLE 12.1
Classification of scoliosis curves by part of the spine affected

Curve type	Apex location
Cervical	C1–C6
Cervicothoracic	C7–T1
Thoracic	T2–T11
Thoracolumbar	T12–L1
Lumbar	L2–L4
Lumbosacral	L5–S1

programmes have reported 1%–3% of teenagers with AIS (Leaver et al. 1982, Goldberg et al. 1995), and in the UK the single largest group with a spinal deformity is progressive AIS, with a reported incidence of 2 per 1000 children (Thompson 2001). Studies from screening programmes, which may detect more cases than otherwise attend clinics, report that structural curves >20° occur in 1–3 per 1000 children (Cassella and Hall 1991). This is clinically significant, as 20° of curvature has historically been a threshold beyond which orthotic intervention is considered. Data collated by Nachemson and Peterson (1995) showed increasing magnitude of curvature with decreasing prevalence (Table 12.2a) (Lonstein 1978). The relationship of the curve magnitude to the male:female ratio, as shown in (Table 12.2b), shows the proportional changes that occur with increasing magnitude (Rogala et al. 1978).

TABLE 12.2a
The association between prevalence and magnitude of curve shows
that smaller deformities are more common than larger deformities

Magnitude of curvature	Prevalence
>10°	2%–3%
>20°	0.3%–0.5%
>30°	0.2%–0.3%

TABLE 12.2b
The association between sex and magnitude of curve reveals that girls have larger scoliosis

Magnitude of curvature	Ratio female:male
6°–10°	1:1
11°–20°	1.4:1
>21°	5.4:1
Curves being treated	7.2:1

Clinical examination

The assessment of children with scoliosis should include the following procedures (Grossman et al. 1995, Taft and Francis 2003):

- observation of any trunk asymmetry in the coronal or sagittal planes, such as shoulder-level obliquity, scapula or rib prominence, waist asymmetry or any other anatomical abnormalities or prominences
- examination of the symmetry at the levels of the anterior and posterior–superior iliac spines and the iliac crests, specifically noting any pelvic obliquity. Any leg-length discrepancy should be determined as this will either cause pelvic obliquity or be accommodated by unilateral hip and knee flexion in the longer leg
- estimation of the alignment of the head over sacrum or any deviation from the midline using a plumb line dropped down from the spinous process of C7; a small weight tied to a cord can be used to visualize the plumb line
- asking the child to bend forward will accentuate any rotational deformity; this can be measured using a 'scoliometer', which works like a spirit level
- asking the child to bend sideways assesses the flexibility of the spine and indicates the extent to which corrective forces can be applied to reduce the curves.

Further examination of the structure of the curves requires radiographic investigation, usually posterior–anterior (PA) and sagittal-view X-rays taken while the child is standing. Lateral-bending PA films can be used to determine the flexibility of the curves. These X-rays will allow measurement of the Cobb angle (Fig. 12.1) and give an indication of vertebral

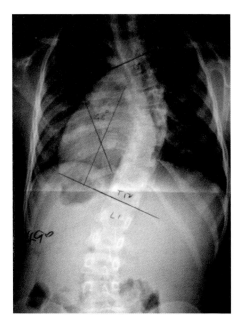

Fig. 12.1 The Cobb angle is measured between the two most inclined vertebrae.

rotation using the grading of pedicle rotation from 0 to 4 (Nash and Moe 1969). X-ray films also provide a means to estimate the level of skeletal maturity using the Risser technique (Risser 1958). The iliac apophysis is graded from 0 to 5, with Risser grade 5 indicating full fusion of the apophysis that correlates with the end of height growth. The risk of curve progression is increased for younger children, lower Risser signs and larger curves (Lonstein and Carlson 1984). For infantile scoliosis the amount of apical vertebral rotation and the rib–vertebra angle difference (RVAD) may differentiate between curves that can resolve and those that may progress (Mehta 1972).

Other assessment techniques that can be used are moiré surface topography (Koepfler 1983), such as the integrated shape imaging system (ISIS) (Turner-Smith 1988), or magnetic resonance imaging (MRI). Investigation with MRI is recommended for children under 12 years of age, as a significant number have been found to have an underlying neuroanatomical abnormality (Evans et al. 1996).

Orthotic management

The realistic objective of orthotic intervention is to prevent or reduce the rate of curve progression rather than to achieve full correction (Willers et al. 1993, Rowe et al. 1997). This serves to delay or prevent the need for surgery. Therefore, while the Cobb angle may be reduced during treatment, curves can be expected to return to their original magnitude, with any permanent correction considered a bonus (Katz 2003).

For a spinal orthosis to be indicated for the treatment of idiopathic scoliosis, protocols may vary but generally follow the regime shown in Table 12.3 (Rowe 2002). Orthotic intervention is typically considered for children with curves ranging from 25° to 45° with Risser sign 0–2 (Emans 1986, Lonstein and Winter 1994). Other factors influencing the use of orthoses would be family history of the condition and also the motivation and willingness of the child and family to follow a strict treatment regimen. Use of most orthoses is advocated for 23 hours per day, while time out of the orthoses is recommended for sports or similar activities. It has been suggested that if full-time compliance is achieved in the first 9 months, the daily regimen can be reduced to 16–18 hours without compromising its efficacy (Emans et al. 1986, Nachemson and Peterson 1995). It is also worth emphasising that the 'quality' of use, the orthosis being positioned correctly and straps fastened to an

TABLE 12.3
Treatment recommendations for scoliosis according to Cobb angle and riser stage

Risser grade	Cobb angle value	Treatment
0–1	0°–20°	Observation
0–1	20°–40°	Orthosis
2–3	0°–30°	Observe
2–3	30°–40°	Orthosis
0–3	40°–50°	Variable options
0–4	>50°	Surgery

From Rowe (2002)

appropriate tightness, is as influential for the efficacy of the treatment as the 'quantity' of time the orthosis is worn. In general, the longer the orthosis is worn correctly, the better the outcome is likely to be (Lou et al. 2004).

Compliance with wearing a spinal orthosis can be a problem for all children and particularly challenging for adolescents because of the overt aesthetic implications. The factors that influence orthotic compliance are a negative body-image, low self-esteem, reduction in participating in social activities and any sleeping problems when wearing an orthosis at night (Lindeman and Behm 1999, Danielsson et al. 2001). Other factors that create stress are the initial bracing period, and any soreness, skin irritation, breathing or eating difficulties, torn clothing, and discomfort during physical activities (MacLean et al. 1989). Studies have shown that compliance is normally much lower than the advocated prescribed time (DiRaimondo and Green 1988). One alternative to the 23 hour per day programme is a night-time only regimen such as the Charleston system (Allington and Bowen 1996, Price et al. 1997). For curvatures of less than 35° such part-time regimens are considered by some to be a more realistic treatment option (Katz & Durrani 2001). Part-time or night-time orthotic regimens may possibly resolve the compliance issues without compromising the effectiveness of intervention, as some results are reported to be consistent with full-time use (Allington and Bowen 1996, Price et al. 1997). At the present time, however, the Scoliosis Research Society still recommends a 23-hour regimen, based on the findings of a meta-analysis (Rowe et al. 1997).

Successful treatment using spinal orthoses can also be influenced by any back pain, respiratory problems or skin breakdown. When back pain is reported, it needs to be considered whether this is due to pathology in the spine, is caused by the orthosis, or is a psychosocial complication (Gunnoe 1990, Ramirez 1999). In principle, respiratory function should not be affected by a correctly fitting orthosis (Korovessis et al. 1996); however, inevitably, the wearing of a rigid, tight-fitting orthosis can result in some restriction of lung function at rest and during exercise (Refsum et al. 1990). This effect is rapidly reversed following orthosis discontinuation, so any reported difficulties from tightness should be relieved by orthosis modification. Concern over skin tolerance to orthosis pressure requires careful management with temporary skin discoloration to be expected (Watts 1979). Bone density in the spine and pelvis is thought not to be affected by orthotic management (Snyder et al. 1995).

Quality of life and related psychosocial outcomes are very important for these children and adolescents. To reduce any adverse psychosocial impact, the orthosis with the lowest effect on quality of life should be considered (Climent and Sanchez 1999). However, it has been shown that quality-of-life outcomes for children treated with spinal orthoses were no lower than in those whose curves were simply observed (Ugwonali et al. 2004). At longer-term follow-up it has also been shown that operative patients had a more negative body image than those who had orthoses (Noonan et al. 1997). A new condition-specific instrument for measuring quality of life outcomes is the Scoliosis Quality of Life Index questionnaire, which has shown to be a valid and reliable assessment of the psychosocial aspects of AIS patients (Feise et al. 2005).

Types of orthosis

The remainder of this chapter describes the various different designs of orthosis that may be considered when orthotic intervention is indicated. Spinal orthoses use the nomenclature of CTLSO, TLSO or LSO depending on which sections of the spine they encompass. Spinal orthoses can be broadly classified into two groups: those that are intended to match and oppose the deforming forces, and those that aim to overcorrect. For both types, corrective forces are applied just below the apex of the curve in the coronal plane, and similarly in the sagittal and transverse planes. The choice of orthosis generally depends upon the experience and preferences of the orthopaedic specialist and orthotist at individual centres. The most commonly used orthoses are discussed in detail here, and other new or less common designs are mentioned briefly towards the end of the chapter.

CUSTOM THORACOLUMBAR–SACRAL ORTHOSIS (TLSO)

A negative plaster-cast mould of the child is needed in order to make a custom TLSO. The cast can be taken whilst the child is either standing or supine. The standing method usually requires using a frame that includes a halter positioned under mandible and occiput to distract and reduce axial loading on the spine (Table 12.3). Alternatively, simply asking the child to lie supine removes the deforming force caused by gravity and enables the spine to be manipulated more easily during the casting process. The results using TLSOs manufactured from the two methods are considered equivalent in controlling the Cobb angle (Wong et al. 2003).

Flexing the child's hips and knees decreases the lumbar lordosis, unlocking the intervertebral facet joints, which renders the spine more flexible and amenable to correction. The cast is moulded to flatten the abdomen to assist lumbar lordosis reduction and to define any bony prominences such as ASIS. The iliac crests are clearly defined to create an exaggerated waistline superior to the iliac crests (Fig. 12.2). This ensures that the TLSO will be securely positioned around the pelvis.

The X-ray is used as a blueprint for orthosis design (Fig. 12.3). The negative cast is filled with plaster of Paris (POP) to create a positive model of the trunk. The positive cast is then modified by adding plaster over prominent bony prominences such as ASIS, iliac crest and inferior rib margins. Conversely, plaster is removed over softer areas such as buttocks and abdomen to create a well-fitting orthosis. Plaster can also be removed to increase correction, in which case additions are then necessary to create voids for the trunk to move into (Fig. 12.4).

The trim-lines of the orthosis are kept as long as is practical to provide the optimum leverage, and areas of high pressure should be avoided by maximizing the area of the orthosis–skin interface. Normal practice aims to obtain 50% reduction of curvature in the orthosis (Emans et al. 1986, Lonstein and Winter 1994). This can be quantified by an 'in-orthosis' X-ray to measure the efficacy of the orthosis, and then with repeated 'out-of-orthosis' X-rays during the treatment period (Fig. 12.5). Showing the family an X-ray of the child in the orthosis, and thereby demonstrating that wearing the orthosis really does reduce the curve may encourage compliance. The in-orthosis X-ray should also be assessed with respect to 'trunk shift' and 'decompensation'. Trunk shift describes how the

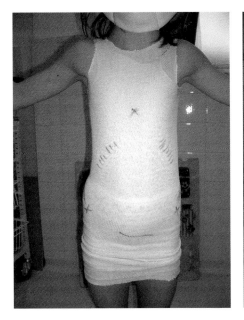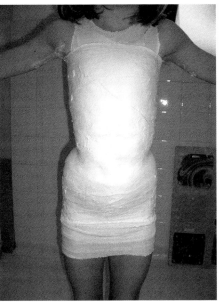

Fig. 12.2 Casting for a TLSO in a standing position using neck halter to create distraction.

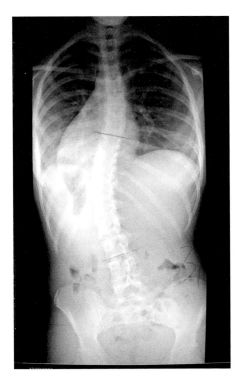

Fig. 12.3 Posterior–anterior viewed X-ray is used to create the blueprint for the TLSO.

145

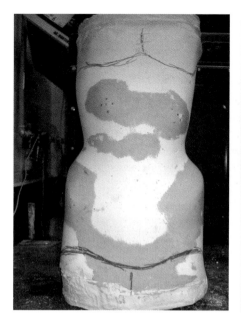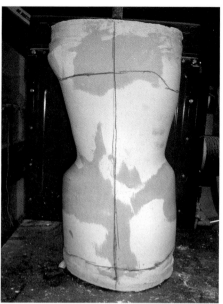

Fig. 12.4 The modified positive cast is modified to accentuate waist and rim of the pelvis and then smoothed; the trim lines are added prior to moulding the plastic.

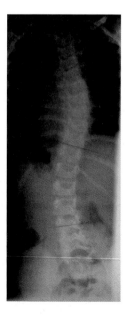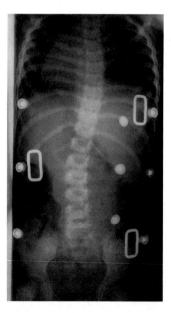

Fig. 12.5 Posterior–anterior X-ray taken in the orthosis (indicated by metal buckles and rivets) and out of orthosis shows the curve reduction achieved partially by controlling pelvic obliquity and application of corrective forces.

asymmetrical body moves towards the midline, so the centre of body weight is over the sacrum. Decompensation is the horizontal distance between vertical lines bisecting the sacrum and the highest vertebral body seen on a standing antero-posterior X-ray (Rudiel and Renshaw 1983).

Custom TLSOs are commonly manufactured from 3 mm or 4.5 mm polypropylene or sub-ortholene to create a rigid cylindrical shell; they may include a lining of polyethylene foam. Spinal orthoses can be made to open either at the front or back, and are secured by fastening straps (Figs 12.6, 12.7). The tightness of the secured orthosis is very important, as is ensuring that strap tension and pad placement are correlated to enhance biomechanical effectiveness (Wong et al. 2000). Anterior trim-lines normally extend from the xyphoid process, below the breast tissue, to the symphysis pubis, and should be shaped adequately over the thighs to allow the hips to flex fully when seated. The posterior trim-lines usually extend from the inferior angle of the scapula to the apex of the buttocks. However, each orthosis will be specifically designed depending on the curve and pattern of the individual child and the nature of their scoliosis. Curvatures of 25°–45° are normally treated up to a maximum apex level of vertebrae T7 using TLSOs. A cervical TLSO (CTLSO) extending to the neck would be required to treat for any deformity above this level and include a metal superstructure, such as those described below in the section on the Milwaukee orthosis.

A custom TLSO may also be used to control significant thoracic kyphosis (Fig. 12.8), sometimes referred to as Scheuermann's disease. The anterior corrective forces need to be applied as high as possible on the chest, by controlling the pelvis (Fig. 12.9), and the posterior force is applied just below the apex of the kyphosis.

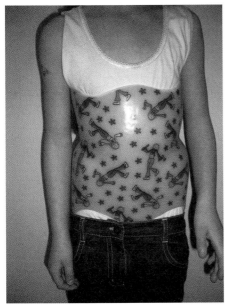

Fig. 12.6 Custom TLSO (anterior view).

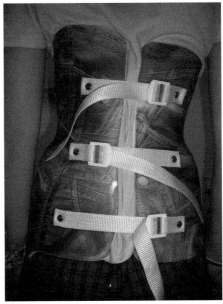

Fig. 12.7 Custom TLSO (posterior view).

147

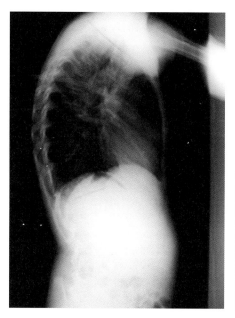 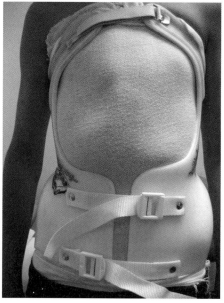

Fig. 12.8 Lateral x-ray showing an excessive thoracic kyphosis, sometimes referred to as Scheuermann's disease.

Fig. 12.9 Another view of custom TLSO prescribed to counter excessive thoracic kyphosis. Note the well-moulded pelvic section, encouraging an anterior tilt and high superior trim-lines under the clavicles; these forces counter the posteriorly applied force just below the apex of the kyphosis.

BOSTON BRACE

The Boston 'brace' system was initially proposed in 1971 as a more cosmetically acceptable low-profile orthosis than its predecessors (Hall et al. 1975, Watts et al. 1977). The orthosis consists of a symmetrical prefabricated TLSO module that is available in a range of standard sizes, or alternatively made to order. The appropriate size is determined by taking measurements at xyphoid, waist, ASIS and hip level. The modules are made of a rigid high-density polypropylene shell with a polyethylene foam lining. A degree of lumbar flexion and abdominal concavity is incorporated to flatten the lumbar lordosis. Lordosis of 15° is the generally accepted optimum value (Olafsson et al. 1995). There are a range of shaped supplementary pads that can be added to allow the modules to be individually customized to meet the biomechanical objectives. Before the module is modified, a blueprint for the design is created using the X-ray. The blueprint is used to plan the length of the orthosis, the trim-lines, pad-placement position and areas of relief (Fig. 12.10). The manufacturers' manuals recommend specific designs for the most common curve patterns.

The Boston system is recommended for scoliosis with Cobb angles of 20°–40° with 50% flexibility of the reduction. This flexibility is important to achieve optimum correction within the orthosis. If there is less flexibility then the system is unlikely to succeed (Emans

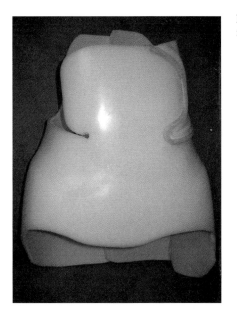

Fig. 12.10 Boston brace TLSO produced by modifying a standard module.

et al. 1986). The recommended regimen involves the orthosis being worn 23 hours per day. The standard module can be trimmed for any of the common curve patterns, up to an apex at a level of T7. The Boston system requires a simultaneous and coordinated physiotherapy programme that encourages children to alter their own posture actively by moving away from the pressure applied by the orthosis. Physiotherapy may help to over-come any hip-flexor tightness and minimize trunk weakness or stiffness incurred by using the orthosis.

A weaning-in period of 2 weeks is recommended, with regular follow-up appointments to ensure correct fit and comfort, with appropriate modifications or replacement of the modules as the child grows. The Boston system has been shown to be somewhat effective for the management of idiopathic scoliosis (Emans et al. 1986, Fernandez-Feliberti et al. 1995). Part-time use may be sufficient when treating small curves; however, full-time use is recommended to prevent the progression of large-magnitude curvatures (Wiley et al. 2000). It is important that the orthotist indicates how tightly the straps need to be fastened by marking the straps and that this is adhered to, together with duration of wear, to ensure the best chance of meeting the treatment objectives (Lou et al. 2004).

MILWAUKEE BRACE

The Milwaukee brace is a CTLSO consisting of a custom-made pelvic girdle with a metal superstructure; the brace was originally developed in 1946 for postoperative applications, but became popular for use in the non-operative treatment of scoliosis from the mid-1950s (Blount and Moe 1973). The orthosis has been used to treat a variety of single, double and triple curve patterns at various levels.

A plaster-cast is required for moulding the pelvic section, together with measurements for the height of the superstructure. The pelvic section was originally made of leather, but these days is usually plastic. The metal superstructure consists of one anterior and two posterior metal uprights fixed to the pelvic section. These extend to anterior submandibular pads and posterior occipital pads that aim to create distractive forces between the head and pelvis. These pads were replaced with a lower-profile neck ring in an effort to make the orthosis less unsightly and to prevent iatrogenically induced mandibular deformities. The objective of the ring is to stimulate and encourage the child to pull away from the contact points thus using muscle power to correct the curvature (Blount and Moe 1973). Pads and straps are added to the metal superstructure to apply corrective forces below the apices of the curvatures. Any lumbar pads can be fitted inside the pelvic section. The advantage of the Milwaukee system is that curvatures with an apex above T7 can be treated, and it is the only choice for high thoracic curves (Lonstein and Winter 1994). A young patient with a large thoracic curve that is at the highest risk of progression maybe best managed by a well-fitting CTLSO (Patwardhan et al. 1996). The protocol is for this orthosis to be worn 23 hours per day, again with the aim of having 50% reduction of the curvatures while wearing the orthosis. The Milwaukee system has shown results that compare favourably with other orthoses (Rowe et al. 1997); although the prognosis for larger curves at a young age remains as low as other orthoses (Lonstein and Winter 1994). However, children may have trouble tolerating this imposing design of orthosis, which stretches from pelvis to throat, and the practical and psychosocial difficulties resulting from this may be seen as a limitation.

CHENEAU ORTHOSIS
The Cheneau custom-made TLSO was designed in Europe, with an emphasis on countering rotational deformities. The orthosis uses laterally applied forces for active correction to work in all three dimensions (Matussek et al. 2000). The design of the orthosis takes account of the surface topography, such as rib humps or vertebral rotations. A plaster-cast is taken in a standing position using a special frame to control lumbar lordosis and trunk stability. The positive cast is radically modified to achieve the desired corrective forces. Where plaster is removed for curve correction an opposite area has additions made to create voids in the orthosis. This is to allow the trunk space to move within the orthosis and to allow for rib expansion on breathing. The orthosis is made from polypropylene or high-density polyethylene and usually is padded over pressure areas or bony prominences. It has an anterior opening with high anterior proximal trim-lines to encourage thoracic extension. The other trim-lines can be varied according to the requirements of the curve pattern being treated. A modified version of this orthosis, which aims for overcorrection, is used more often (Weiss et al. 2002).

Early reports suggested that the Cheneau orthosis achieved up to 41% in brace correction (Hopf and Heine 1985). Imaging suggests that the Cheneau is able to reduce the mean thoracic Cobb angle significantly (Schmitz et al. 2005). The amount of primary correction is again of importance, particularly for the overcorrection of the modified Cheneau. It has been suggested that the Cheneau orthosis is more effective than other orthoses in decreasing spinal decompensation (Von Diemling et al. 1995), and more effective than other rigid orthotic systems in controlling progression (Wong and Liu 2003). Use of the Cheneau orthosis has been found to prevent Cobb angle progression (Rigo et al. 2002) and, in combination with an intensive rehabilitation programme, has reduced the need for surgery (Weiss et al. 2002).

WILMINGTON ORTHOSIS

The Wilmington orthosis was developed as a more attractive alternative to the Milwaukee brace and was designed by MacEwen in 1969 (Bunnell et al. 1980). It is in fact a custom-made TLSO but incorporates several key design features. The cast is taken with the child lying supine on a special table which permits the maximum corrective forces to be applied during the measurement process. An X-ray is taken with the patient in the cast to determine the magnitude of curve reduction. The orthosis is usually fabricated from polypropylene with an anterior overlapping opening secured by fastening straps. As with other types of TLSO, treatment with the Wilmington is indicated for curves of between 25° and 40° with an apex below T7. Usage is recommended full time, 23 hours per day, but satisfactory results may be achieved with just 16 hours per day (Allington and Bowen 1996). After the patient has been wearing the orthosis for 1 month, an X-ray is taken within the orthosis to confirm that the amount of curve reduction is maintained. X-rays are repeated at 6-monthly intervals, out of the orthosis, until the weaning-out period at skeletal maturity. The Wilmington orthosis has been shown to be effective and can alter the natural history of idiopathic curves of 40° or less (Basset et al. 1986, Allington and Bowen 1996).

CHARLESTON ORTHOSIS

Nocturnal regimens have been proposed to overcome the psychosocial problems and compliance issues encountered when TLSOs are used in the daytime. The Charleston 'bending brace' has been a prescribed as a night-time treatment since the late 1970s (Price et al. 1990), and continues to be favoured in some centres (Katz et al. 1997). The orthosis is produced from a plaster-cast taken with the patient standing. An X-ray is used as a blueprint to modify the cast appropriately where it is important to decide which curve is the primary one, as this is the curve that is attempted to be 'unbent'. A Charleston brace consists of a rigid plastic polypropylene shell with a foam liner. The trim-lines are more radical than other TLSOs in that they are extended longer on the concave side of the curve and shortened on the convex side. The TLSO does not have to be trimmed to allow sitting or standing as the orthosis is only used supine. The orthosis has an anterior opening with fastening straps to securely tighten and apply greater corrective forces. The principle is that the scoliosis curves are reduced by overcorrection produced by opposite lateral bending forces. The orthosis is fitted in the supine position with an initial in-orthosis X-ray taken to confirm the amount of correction achieved. An accompanying exercise programme is recommended to maintain or increase muscle strength, flexibility and promote postural alignment (Hooper et al. 2003).

PROVIDENCE ORTHOSIS

The Providence orthosis has been used since 1992 (D'Amato et al. 2001). The orthosis was developed when it was observed that significant overcorrection of scoliosis curves could be achieved using an acrylic frame to apply corrective forces. The frame was originally developed to assess spine flexibility for preoperative radiographic planning. The patient is clinically evaluated and assessed, and is then positioned on a polycarbonate measurement and casting board. Information from a standing X-ray is then used as a guide to position bolsters on the board using a grid of surface holes. This allows accurate application of corrective lateral forces to the patient's body. Originally all patients were removed from the board then had a wrap plaster-cast applied, and returned to the board for bolsters to be repositioned whilst the plaster was allowed to set.

It is proposed that in around 95% of cases, however, computers can be used to manufacture the orthoses, just using digitized measurements from the polycarbonate board. The orthosis is manufactured from polypropylene to the measurements or to the cast. Trim-lines for the orthosis are designed to apply appropriate correction with extended material on the concave side of the curves and shortened on convex. The orthosis is anterior-opening, with securing fastening straps, and corrective straps can also be fitted if required. More recent developments have used carbon-fibre reinforcements in the Providence orthosis. This aims to prevent the plastic from distorting and to allow void cut-out areas to make the orthosis cooler and more comfortable. The Providence orthosis is fitted in the supine position. A pressure-sensitive film is used to monitor the amount of corrective force to avoid any created excessive pressures. This can also be used to measure effectiveness during growth.

The Providence orthosis is thought to achieve an average in-brace correction of 96%, with the more flexible thoracolumbar and lumbar curves being overcorrected as viewed by X-ray (D'Amato et al. 2001). Although the orthosis can be prescribed for higher apices and curve values, it is most suitable for treating flexible curves under 35° and with the primary curve apex below T8 (D'Amato et al. 2001).

The use of night-time orthoses has the advantage that greater correction of the scoliosis curves can be achieved in the orthosis, as they do not need to be tolerated in an upright position. The placement of forces is not limited by the requirement of having the iliac crest as the most distal point of corrective force application, and the head does not have to be maintained over the pelvis. Therefore placement of these forces allows greater in-brace correction up to 100% or more for primary curves (Price et al. 1997, D'Amato et al. 2001).

Proponents of the system suggest that the results of part-time or night-time orthoses are comparable to full-time regimens (Bowen et al. 2001), with up to 74% of progression halted (D'Amato et al. 2001). It has been reported that curves up to 40° respond as well to part-time as to full-time orthoses (Frederico and Renshaw 1990). Single curves may respond best to night-time only treatment, but patient selection requires care (Katz et al. 1997, Trivedi and Thompson 2001). A combination of night and day orthoses may be used if progression is observed on curves over 35° with high apices (D'Amato et al. 2001).

Two relatively recent innovations can be classified as more 'flexible' spinal orthoses in comparison to the rigid systems already described. Compliance is proposed to be better with these systems than with rigid orthoses as they are less bulky and restrictive and allow greater body movement within the orthosis. SpineCor was developed in the mid-1990s to treat curves of 15°–30° (Coillard et al. 1999) and treatment of curves as low as 10° have also been advocated; these are children who would not normally be treated using rigid orthoses. The SpineCor orthosis consists of a plastic pelvic girdle held in position by thigh and crotch straps and a fabric corset on the torso. Elastic straps are attached to the girdle and wrapped around the body to create the corrective forces and reduce scoliosis. The orthosis aims to induce progressive postural changes and correction of curves during normal daily activities (Coillard et al. 1999). Assessment requires a computerized digital mapping system that evaluates postural geometry by creating a 3-dimensional representation of the body. This is then used in the prescription decision and orthosis-fitting process. The advocates of SpineCor recommend that it is worn full time, and they claim that it has the advantage of preserving normal body movement while also being worn easily under regular clothing. The SpineCor system is said to prevent curve progression and even to reduce curves (Rivard et al. 2000, Smith 2002), although these curves tend to be smaller than those treated by other systems. A cohort of patients treated by the developers demonstrated a decrease in curvature in the orthosis, followed by correction or stabilization in a 2-year follow-up (Coillard et al. 2003). Long-term follow-up to evaluate the orthosis is still required, although there have been some studies comparing them with rigid orthoses (Weiss and Weiss 2005).

The TriaC system was developed in the Netherlands as an alternative to conventional orthoses (Veldhuizen et al. 2002). The orthosis is an open system that applies corrective lateral forces, and is described as applying anterior progression force counteracted by a posterior force and torque (Veldhuizen et al. 2002). The TriaC orthosis comprises lumbar and thoracic components connected by a framework of metal rods, plastic parts, spiral springs and fabric straps. The hinged elements allow motion whilst maintaining the application of a continuous level of corrective force. Like the SpineCor system, the TriaC orthosis aims to offer high comfort and acceptable appearance, and to be less restrictive than more rigid designs; the TriaC is similarly advocated for smaller curves that would not otherwise be treated using plastic TLSOs, making comparisons of effectiveness difficult (Veldhuizen et al. 2002).

Other non-surgical treatments for scoliosis include physical exercise, postural feedback and electrical stimulation. Physical exercise treatment is based on the theory that unbalanced muscle tone is a cause of scoliosis and that simply exercising can therefore help to reduce the deformity (Weiss 1992, Mooney et al. 2000). There is no fixed protocol for the exercises but programmes are based on improving the power of the paraspinal muscles which can contribute to straightening the spine (Wong and Liu 2003). Physical exercise may help to reduce unbalanced muscle tone, but these techniques should generally be used in conjunction with orthoses (Wong and Liu 2003).

Posture monitoring is an electronic training device that uses the principle of a learned physiological response (Dworkin 1982). A subsequent device called Micro Straight has been evaluated, with promising results, and has been found to be well tolerated (Wong et al. 2001). The device is fitted such that when incorrect posture occurs, an audible tone sounds until the patient adopts the corrected posture. Lasting improvement might in theory be achieved through strengthening muscles and increasing postural awareness; however, a long-term study would be required before this treatment could be recommended (Wong et al. 2001).

Surface electrical stimulation has been used since the 1970s and is often referred to as lateral electrical surface stimulation (LESS) (Axelgaard and Brown 1983), when applied to lateral muscles, or electro-spinal orthosis (ESO) (McCollough 1986) when applied to paraspinal muscles. This treatment has not been widely accepted or continued due to studies showing poor results (Durham et al. 1990, Bertrand et al. 1992), and conventional orthotic treatment seems to be more effective (Rowe et al. 1997, Bowen et al. 2001).

Conclusion

Currently it is difficult to make any clear comparisons between the efficacy of the various types of orthoses because of different prescription criteria and the heterogeneity of children's conditions. Some optimal parameters have been established so that future studies can be more rigorous in making valid and reliable comparisons in the future (Richards et al. 2005). On balance, to date, rigid orthoses can be regarded as the most effective nonoperative intervention for moderate idiopathic scoliosis (Wong and Liu 2003). That said, because of the difficult life issues faced by children and adolescents with scoliosis, the most appropriate treatment will be the one that will be a balance of best outcome, greatest comfort and acceptable cosmesis (Patwardhan et al. 1996).

References

Allington NJ, Bowen JR (1996) Adolescent idiopathic scoliosis: treatment with the Wilmington Brace; a comparison of full and part time use. *J Bone Joint Surg Am* **78**: 1056–61.

Axelgaard J, Brown JC (1983) Lateral electrical stimulation for the treatment of progressive idiopathic scoliosis. *Spine* **8**: 242–60.

Bertrand SL, Drvaric DM, Lange N, Lucas PR, Deutsch SD, Herndon JH, Roberts JM (1992) Electrical stimulation for idiopathic scoliosis. *Clin Orthop* **276**: 176–81.

Blount WP, Moe JH (1973) *The Milwaukee Brace*. Baltimore: Williams & Wilkins.

Bowen JR, Keeler KA, Pelegie S (2001) Adolescent idiopathic scoliosis managed by a nighttime bending brace. *Orthopedics* **24**: 967–70.

Bradford DS, Lonstein JE, Moe JH, Ogilvie JW, Winter RB (1987) *Moe's Textbook of Scoliosis and Other Spinal Deformities*, 2nd edn. Philadelphia: W.B. Saunders.

Bunnell WP, MacEwen GD, Jayakumar S (1980) The use of plastic jackets in the non-operative treatment of idiopathic scoliosis: preliminary report. *J Bone Joint Surg Am* **62**: 31–8.

Burgoyne W, Fairbank J (2001) The management of scoliosis. *Current Paediatrics* **11**: 323–31.

Cassella MC, Hall JE (1991) Current treatment approaches in the non-operative and operative management of adolescent idiopathic scoliosis. *Phys Ther* **71**: 897–909.

Climent JM, Sanchez J (1999) Impact of the type of brace on the quality of life of adolescents with spine deformities. *Spine* **24**: 1903–8.

Cobb JR (1948) Outline for the study of scoliosis. *Instr Course Lect* **5**: 261–75.

Coillard C, Leroux MA, Zabjek KF, Rivard CH (1999) The reducibility of idiopathic scoliosis during non-operative treatment. *Ann Chir* **53**: 781–91.

Coillard C Leroux MA, Zabjek KF, Rivard CH (2003) SpineCor a non rigid brace for the treatment of idiopathic scoliosis: post treatment results. *Eur Spine J* **12**: 141–8.

D'Amato CR, Griggs S, McCoy B (2001) Nighttime bracing with the Providence brace in adolescent girls with idiopathic scoliosis. *Spine* **26**: 2006–12.

Danielsson AJ, Wiklund I, Pehrsson K, Nachemson AL (2001) Health-related quality of life in patients with adolescent scoliosis: a matched follow-up at least 20 years after treatment with brace or surgery. *Eur Spine J* **10**: 278–88.

DiRaimondo CV, Green NE (1988) Brace-wear compliance in patients with adolescent idiopathic scoliosis. *J Pediatr Orthop* **8**: 143–6.

Dobbs MB, Lenke LG, Morcuende J, Weinstein SL, Bridwell KH, Sponseller PD (2001) Incidence of neural axis abnormalities in infantile patients diagnosed with idiopathic scoliosis; is screening MRI necessary? *Scoliosis Research Society, Paper 10, presented at the 36th Annual Scoliosis Research Society Meeting, Cleveland, Ohio.*

Durham JW, Moskowitz A, Whitney J (1990) Surface electrical stimulation versus brace in treatment of idiopathic scoliosis. *Spine* **15**: 888–92.

Dworkin B (1982) Postural training device. *Health Psychol* **1**: 45–9.

Emans JB, Kaelin A, Bancel P, Hall JE, Miller ME (1986) The Boston bracing system for IS; a follow-up results in 295 patients. *Spine* **11**: 792–801

Evans SC, Edgar MA, Hall-Craggs M, Powell MP, Taylor BA, Noordeen HH (1996) MRI of idiopathic juvenile scoliosis. *J Bone Joint Surg Br* **78**: 314–17.

Feise RJ, Donaldson S, Crowther ER, Menke JM, Wright JG (2005) Construction and validation of the scoliosis quality of life index in adolescent idiopathic scoliosis. *Spine* **30**: 1310–15.

Fernandez-Feliberti R, Flynn J, Ramirez N, Trautmann M, Alegria M (1995) Effectiveness of TLSO bracing in the conservative treatment of AIS. *J Pediatr Orthop* **15**: 176–81.

Frederico DJ, Renshaw TS (1990) Results of treatment of idiopathic scoliosis with the Charleston bending orthosis. *Spine* **15**: 886–7.

Goldberg CJ, Dowling FE, Fogarty EE, Moore DP (1995) Adolescent idiopathic scoliosis as developmental instability. *Genetica* **96**: 247–55.

Grossman TW, Mazur JM, Cummings RJ (1995) An evaluation of the Adams Forward Bend Test and the scoliometer in a scoliosis school screening setting. *J Pediatr Orthop* **15**: 535–8.

Gunnoe BA (1990) Adolescent idiopathic scoliosis. *Orthop Rev* **19**: 35–43.

Hall JE, Miller W, Shurman W, Stanish W (1975) A refined concept in the orthotic management of idiopathic scoliosis. *Prosthet Orthot Int* **29**: 7–13.

Hooper CR, Reed FE, Price CT (2003) The Charleston bending brace: an orthotist's guide to scoliosis management. www.srs.org

Hopf C, Heine J (1985) Long-term results of the conservative treatment of scoliosis using the Cheneau brace. *Z Orthop Ihre Grenzgeb* **123**: 312–22.

Katz DE, Richards S, Browne RH, Herring JA (1997) A comparison between the Boston brace and the Charleston bending brace in adolescent idiopathic scoliosis. *Spine* **22**: 1302–12.

Katz DE, Durrani AA (2001) Factors that influence outcome in bracing large curves in patients with adolescent idiopathic scoliosis. *Spine* **26**: 2354–61.

Katz DE (2003) The etiology and natural history of idiopathic scoliosis. *J Prosthet Orthot* **15** (suppl.): 3–9.

Koepfler JW (1983) Moiré topography in medicine. *J Biol Photogr* **51**: 3–9.

Korovessis P, Filos KS, Georgopoulos D (1996) Long-term alterations of respiratory function in adolescents wearing a brace for idiopathic scoliosis. *Spine* **21**: 1979–84.

Leaver JM, Alvik A, Warren MD (1982) Prescriptive screening for adolescent idiopathic scoliosis: a review of the evidence. *Int J Epidemiol* **11**: 101–11.

Lindeman M, Behm K (1999) Cognitive strategies and self-esteem as predictors of brace-wear compliance in patients with idiopathic scoliosis and kyphosis. *J Pediatr Orthop* **19**: 493–9.

Lonstein JE (1978) Risk of progression of idiopathic scoliosis in skeletally immature patients. *Spine: State of the Art Reviews* **1**: 181–93.

Lonstein JE, Carlson JM (1984) The prediction of curve progression in untreated idiopathic scoliosis during growth. *J Bone Joint Surg Am* **66**: 1061–71.

Lonstein JE, Winter RB (1994) The Milwaukee brace for the treatment of adolescent idiopathic scoliosis: a review of one thousand and twenty patients. *J Bone Joint Surg Am* **76**: 1207–21.

155

Lou E, Raso VJ, Hill DL, Mahood JK, Moreau MJ (2004) Correlation between quantity and quality of orthosis wear and treatment outcomes in adolescent idiopathic scoliosis. *Prosthet Orthot Int* **28**: 49–54.

Lowe TG, Edgar M, Margulies JY, Raso VJ, Rivard C (2000) Current concepts review. Etiology of idiopathic scoliosis: current trends in research. *J Bone Joint Surg Am* **82**: 1157–65

MacLean WE, Green NE, Pierre CB, Ray DC (1989) Stress and coping with scoliosis: psychological effects on adolescents and their families. *J Pediatr Orthop* **9**: 257–61.

Matussek J, Mellerowicz H, Klockner C, Sauerlandt B, Nahr K, Neff G (2000) Two and three dimensional correction of scoliosis by corset treatment. Optimized conservative therapy of idiopathic scoliosis with the improved Cheneau corset. *Orthopäde* **29**: 490–9.

McCollough NC (1986) Non-operative treatment of idiopathic scoliosis using electrical surface stimulation. *Spine* **11**: 802–4.

Mehta MH (1972) The rib–vertebra angle in the early diagnosis between resolving and progressive infantile scoliosis. *J Bone Joint Surg Br* **54**: 230–43.

Moe JH, Bradford DS, Winter RB, Lonstein JE (1978) *Scoliosis and Other Spinal Deformities*. Philadelphia: W.B. Saunders.

Mooney V, Gulick J, Pozos R (2000) A preliminary report on the effect of measured strength training in adolescent scoliosis. *J Spinal Disord* **13**: 102–7.

Nachemson AL, Peterson LE (1995) Effectiveness of treatment with a brace in girls who have adolescent idiopathic scoliosis. *J Bone Joint Surg Am* **77**: 815–22.

Nash CL, Moe JE. (1969) A study of vertebral rotation. *J Bone Joint Surg Am* **51**: 223–9.

Noonan KJ, Dolan LA, Jacobson WC, Weinstein SL (1997) Long-term psychosocial characteristics of patients treated for idiopathic scoliosis. *J Pediatr Orthop* **17**: 712–17.

Olafsson Y, Saraste H, Soderlund V, Hoffsten M (1995) Boston brace in the treatment of idiopathic scoliosis. *J Pediatr Orthop* **15**: 524–7.

Patwardhan AG, Gavin TM, Bunch WH, Dvonch VM, Vanderby R, Meade K, Sartori M (1996) Biomechanical comparison of the Milwaukee brace (CTLSO) and the TLSO for treatment of idiopathic scoliosis. *J Prosthet Orthot* **8**: 115–23.

Price CT, Scott DS, Reed FE, Riddick MF (1990) Nighttime bracing for adolescent idiopathic scoliosis with the Charleston bending brace. Preliminary report. *Spine* **15**: 1295–9.

Price CT, Scott DS, Reed FR, Sproul JT, Riddick MF (1997) Nighttime bracing for adolescent idiopathic scoliosis with the Charleston bending brace: long-term follow-up. *J Pediatr Orthop* **17**: 703–7.

Ramirez N, Johnston CE 2nd, Browne RH, Vazquez S (1999) Back pain during orthotic treatment of idiopathic scoliosis. *J Pediatr Orthop* **19**: 198–201.

Refsum HE, Naess-Andresen CF, Lange JE (1990) Pulmonary function and gas exchange at rest and exercise in adolescent girls with mild idiopathic scoliosis during treatment with the Boston Brace. *Spine* **8**: 242–60.

Richards BS, Bernstein RM, D'Amato CR, Thompson GH (2005) Standardization of criteria for adolescent idiopathic scoliosis brace studies: SRS Committee on Bracing and Nonoperative Management. *Spine* **30**: 2068–75.

Rigo M, Quera SG, Puigdevall N, Martinez M (2002) Retrospective results in immature idiopathic scoliotic patients treated with a Cheneau brace. *Stud Health Technol Inform* **88**: 241–5.

Risser JC (1958) The iliac apophysis: an invaluable sign in the management of scoliosis. *Clin Orthop* **11**: 111–19.

Rivard CH, Coillard C, Leroux MA (2000) SpineCor: a new therapeutic approach for idiopathic scoliosis. *J Prosthet Orthot* **10**: 71–6.

Rogala EH, Drummond DS, Gurr J (1978) Scoliosis: incidence and natural history, a prospective epidemiological study. *J Bone Joint Surg Am* **60**: 173–6.

Rowe MF, Adler F, Emans JB, Gardner-Bonneau D (1997) A meta-analysis of the efficacy of non-operative treatments for idiopathic scoliosis. *J Bone Joint Surg Am* **79**: 664–74.

Rowe DE (2002) Non-operative treatment for idiopathic scoliosis. *Scoliosis Research Society CME Course: Fundamentals of Spinal Deformity II, Seattle, WA, September 18.*

Rudicel S, Renshaw TS (1983) The effect of the Milwaukee brace on spinal decompnsation in idiopathic scoliosis. *Spine* **8**: 385–7.

Schmitz A, Konig R, Kandyba J, Pennekamp P, Schmitt O, Jaeger UE (2005) Visualization of the effect on the spinal profile in idiopathic scoliosis. *Eur Spine J* **14**: 138–43.

Smith KM (2002) Elastic strapping orthosis for adolescent idiopathic scoliosis: a preliminary report and initial clinical observations. *J Prosthet Orthot* **14**: 13–18.

156

Snyder BD, Zaltz I, Breitenbach BS, Kido TH, Myers ER, Emans JB (1995) Does bracing affect bone density in adolescent scoliosis? *Spine* **20**: 1554–60.

Taft E, Francis R (2003) Evaluation and management of scoliosis. *J Pediatr Health Care* **17**: 42–4.

Thompson AG (ed.) (2001) *The Management of Spinal Deformity in the United Kingdom; Guide to Practice*. British Scoliosis Society Executive.

Trivedi JM, Thompson JD (2001) Results of Charleston bracing in skeletally immature patients with idiopathic scoliosis. *J Pediatr Orthop* **21**: 277–80.

Turner-Smith AR (1988) A television/computer three-dimensional surface shape measurement system. *J Biomech* **21**: 515–29.

Ugwonali OF, Lomas G, Choe JC, Hyman JE, Lee FY, Vitale MG, Roye DP (2004) Effect of bracing on the quality of life of adolescents with idiopathic scoliosis. *Spine J* **4**: 254–60.

Veldhuizen AG, Cheung J, Bulthuis GJ, Nijenbanning G (2002) A new orthotic device in the non-operative treatment of idiopathic scoliosis. *Med Eng Phys* **24**: 209–18.

Von-Diemling U, Wagner UA, Schmitt O (1995) Long-term effect of brace treatment on spinal decompensation in idiopathic scoliosis. A comparison of Milwaukee brace and Cheneau corset. *Z Orthop Ihre Grenzgeb* **133**: 270–3.

Watts HG, Hall JE, Stanish W (1977) The Boston brace system for the treatment of low thoracic and lumbar scoliosis by the use of a girdle without superstructure. *Clin Orthop* **126**: 87–92.

Watts HG (1979) Bracing in spinal deformities. *Orthop Clin North Am* **10**: 769–85.

Weiss HR (1992) Influence of an in-patient exercise programme on scoliotic curve. *Ital J Orthop Traumatol* **18**: 395–406.

Weiss HR, Weiss G, Schaar HJ (2002) Conservative management in patients with scoliosis – does it reduce the incidence of surgery? *Stud Health Technol Inform* **91**: 342–7.

Weiss HR, Weiss GM (2005) Brace treatment during pubertal growth spurt in girls with idiopathic scoliosis: a prospective trial comparing two different concepts. *Pediatr Rehabil* **8**: 199–206.

Wiley JW, Thomson JD, Mitchell TM, Smith BG, Banta JV (2000) Effectiveness of the Boston brace in the treatment of large curves in AIS. *Spine* **25**: 2326–32.

Willers U, Normelli H, Aaro S, Svensson O, Hedland R (1993) Long-term results of Boston brace treatment on vertebral rotation in AIS. *Spine* **18**: 432–5.

Wong MS, Mak AFT, Luk KDK, Evans JH, Brown B (2000) Effectiveness and biomechanics of spinal orthoses in the treatment of adolescent idiopathic scoliosis. *Prosthet Orthot Int* **24**: 148–62.

Wong MS, Mak AFT, Luk KDK, Evans JH, Brown B (2001) Effectiveness of audio-biofeedback in postural training for adolescent idiopathic scoliosis patients. *Prosthet Orthot Int* **25**: 60–70.

Wong MS, Lee JTC, Luk KDK, Chan LCK (2003) Effect of different casting methods on adolescent idiopathic scoliosis. *Prosthet Orthot Int* **23**: 121–31.

Wong MS, Liu WC (2003) Critical review on non-operative management of adolescent idiopathic scoliosis. *Prosthet Orthot Int* **27**: 242–53.

13
PROTECTIVE AND CORRECTIVE HEADWEAR

Sheila Kellner and Trevor da Silva

Orthoses for the head are commonly referred to as helmets. Helmets are most readily associated with protective applications, but in recent times they have also been used as a corrective treatment for infants with misshapen heads. The first part of this chapter reviews some of the current trends in the prescription of protective helmets. The second part of the chapter describes approaches for the orthotic management of plagiocephaly.

Protective headwear

Protective headwear can be useful in the management of any pathologies and neurodevelopmental conditions where the child is at increased risk of head injury or self-harm. Helmets can be categorized to describe the extent of their coverage of head and face, as well as the degree of impact resistance they offer, that is, hard- or soft-shell designs. Helmets may either be standard sizes that are customized to fit the individual child, or be entirely custom-made.

CLINICAL INDICATIONS

There are few studies which focus on the prevalence of head injuries to children with physical disabilities (Sneed and Stencel 2001). Common conditions for which protective helmets may be prescribed include seizure disorders, self-injurious behaviours, postoperative protection, haemophilia, cerebral palsy, ataxia, dystonia and general unsteadiness (Sneed and Stencel 2001). Many people with these disorders suffer from frequent falls, and are at high risk for severe maxillofacial and head injuries. In addition, there are children who present with head sizes that are unusually large or small; this can restrict safe participation in recreational activities such as cycling or horseback riding that require the use of a helmet, as conventional helmets may not fit properly.

Children who are at increased risk for head injury may be prohibited from attending school or participating in community activities unless they are wearing a protective helmet. The use of a helmet may give the child a more normal level of social and physical interaction and participation. However, these developmental advantages must be balanced with the potentially negative psychological consequences for the child and family of using a piece of equipment that makes them stand out from their peers.

Seizure disorders

Seizure disorders occur with a spectrum of pathologies that most frequently include epilepsy but also have some other neurodevelopmental conditions. Individual seizure patterns vary from child to child; therefore it is important to document the frequency, severity and duration of the seizures as part of the assessment and ongoing review. Furthermore, if possible, it is important to distinguish whether falls resulting from seizures are always in the same direction or multidirectional, as this can influence the design of the helmet. If the child always falls forward, for instance, extra-thick padding can be added to the front to provide additional cushioning to the forehead as well as offering some relief for the nose.

Self-harm

Disturbing self-injurious behaviours include repetitive banging of the head against hard surfaces, often called head-banging; repetitive blows to different parts of the head and face using the fists; or the use of the mouth and teeth for self-mutilation, as seen for example in disorders such as Lesch–Nyhan disease and Pica syndrome. Lesch–Nyhan disease is an X-linked recessive metabolic disorder found almost exclusively in boys. It manifests as psycho-neurological features including compulsive self-mutilation despite having full sensation of pain, and also choreoathetosis, spasticity, and learning disability (Nyhan 1976). Patients who bite their fingers compulsively can be prevented from harming themselves by using a helmet with a face protector, and may potentially be trained out of the habit (Eguchi et al.1994). An alternative is to keep the hands away from the face by constraining the elbows in an extended position using fabric gaiters.

Pica behaviour is characterized by compulsive eating of non-edible substances such as hair, plaster, rope, and flakes of paint. Symptoms may remit during childhood, but occasionally persist into adolescence. There are a variety of strategies to prevent the child eating noxious substances, though there is little evidence to support any one strategy. Helmets with full-face coverage can be prescribed for this population to prevent the wearer any access to their mouth using a hand. Helmets, such as those used for fencing, may achieve this treatment goal very effectively, but this must be balanced against the risk of isolating the child socially and psychologically (McAdam et al. 2004). It is often necessary to secure and fix a clear plastic face-shield or moulded mouth-guard to the front of the helmet. If the child has the dexterity to remove the helmet independently, supplemental restraint orthoses may be required such as elbow gaiters or another orthosis which limits elbow flexion.

Postoperative

Helmets are prescribed following surgery or head trauma to protect the child from further brain injury when the protective role of the skull has been compromised. This may be for only a short period of time or for a longer duration depending on the circumstances. In a craniectomy, a portion of the patient's skull is excised to allow for relief of intracranial pressure due to brain-swelling following stroke or traumatic brain injury. Patients are often required to wear helmets during rehabilitation. The degree of cranial coverage of the helmet is based on the size and location of the skin flap, as well as on the functional status of the patient. In some cases, the excised skull fragment is replaced when the patient's status has stabilized. Greater protection may be required with patients that may have secondary conditions that affect balance and coordination. The duration of helmet use depends on the individual medical and functional status.

Haemophilia
Haemophilia is a blood disorder characterized by a deficiency of coagulation factor VIII. Children with haemophilia are at risk of serious internal haemorrhaging from relatively mild external trauma. Young children in the early stages of learning to stand and walk can have poor balance and coordination and suffer from frequent falls. These infants may be considered candidates for helmets to minimize potential head injuries until their balance and stability are well established.

Ataxia, dystonia and general unsteadiness
Neurodevelopmental conditions that impair coordination and balance, such as cerebral palsy, ataxia or dystonia, are often associated with inconsistent gait deviations. Like other children with general and profound unsteadiness these children may be prescribed helmets since they are at high risk for multidirectional falls. Moreover, children with these conditions may present with head shapes and sizes that are significantly out of proportion. Macrocephaly is characterized by excessive head size. Hydrocephalus is a condition in which there is an accumulation of cerebrospinal fluid within the skull that may be under increased pressure. It is characterized by significant enlargement of the head and a prominent forehead. Microcephaly is characterized by abnormal smallness of the head. Helmets may be prescribed for this population for protection during ambulatory and recreational activities.

ASSESSMENT AND SELECTION OF A SUITABLE PROTECTIVE HELMET
There are three options when selecting a protective helmet: (1) using a commercially available sports helmet, (2) using a standard protective helmet designed specifically for children with disabilities, and (3) making a helmet to fit an individual child. The type of helmet that will be suitable for a particular child depends on several key issues. First, the helmet must be 'fit for purpose', which is largely related to the clinical indication, as described. Helmets are often classified as being either 'hard' or 'soft', depending on the impact resistance provided by the outer shell. Children who fall rarely and are usually only unaided indoors may be adequately served by a softer design, whilst children who charge around independently outside, and who are at risk of falling with greater impact, will require the protection of a hard-shell design. The extent of the head and face to be protected is also part of this design and prescription process. Another key factor is the size and shape of the child's head, which determines whether a standard size can even be considered or whether custom fabrication is necessary. Whilst many children do use standard helmets satisfactorily, without encountering problems, there are several design factors which are worth considering when selecting a helmet design for a child (Ryan et al.1992).

Prefabricated helmets

One option is to purchase a commercially available sports or other type of ready-made helmet, such as those used for hockey, rugby, martial arts (Fig. 13.1) or cycling. These prefabricated helmets are generally designed for people with regular head shapes and for specific activities. Prefabricated helmets are designed for a generic fit, and are usually fitted based solely on a measure of head circumference, although many designs include some minor adjustability. In addition, there are modular designs of helmet which can be assembled and fitted by the orthotist in the clinic, while the patient waits. As we have already recognized, this means that prefabricated designs may not be suitable for children with heads of unusual size or shape. The ventilation slots in many prefabricated sports helmets are designed to conduct the flow of air through the helmet as the wearer moves. This design may not work efficiently for a child whose movements and ambulation patterns may be significantly slower or absent. Inadequate cranial ventilation can reduce wearing compliance due excessive heat retention, and hygiene can become a further complication (Ryan et al. 1992).

The fact that sports helmets are constructed for a specific application often means that they are not always safe or suitable for other purposes. Likewise, orthotists should be careful to point out that their custom-made helmets do not meet the stringent requirements required for approval as, for example, a cycling helmet. For children requiring protection specifically for cycling, therefore, it may be more appropriate to adapt a standard helmet. Notably, however, concerns have been raised that cycling helmets do not always fit their typical user adequately and may be associated with increased risk of head injury even in people without impairments (Rivara et al. 1999).

Typical suspension of prefabricated helmets is achieved using a chin strap, with or without some form of chin cup. Orthodontic problems in growing children have been identified as a result of excessive pressure applied to the chin by the straps to keep the helmet

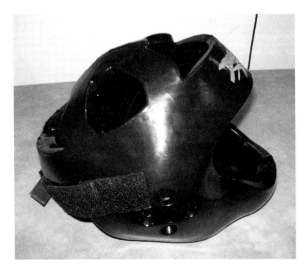

Fig. 13.1 Standard padded helmet used in martial arts.

in place (Ryan et al. 1992). The strap is a crucial part of the design, ensuring that the helmet remains on the child's head in the event of a fall. Inappropriate fit and suspension of the helmet may cause it to rotate or slide off the head, impairing the child's peripheral field of vision and increasing the likelihood of injury. Furthermore, with repetitive use, some commercial helmets may not provide adequate long-term protection due to design parameters which only enable them to withstand a single impact. Weight can also be a factor. Some prefabricated helmets can weigh 2.5 lb or more with any additional hardware such as face shields or wire guards. Despite this, prefabricated helmets are useful in certain circumstances, especially when the head has a regular shape; an example is lightweight soft helmets for infants when the risk of injury is present but low (Fig. 13.2).

Custom-made helmets
When the headwear is made to fit a specific child, a custom-made protective helmet has several clinical and functional advantages over prefabricated designs, including a close fit and a design suited to the risks associated with their favoured activities. Depending on the requirements of the child, and the preferences of the orthotist, the helmet may be of a 'scrum' type (Fig. 13.3), which is made according to specific measurements, or a 'moulded' design. Either design may incorporate additional padding over the more vulnerable areas such as the forehead (if the child often falls forward) or to the posterior aspect (if the child often falls backwards). The custom-moulded helmet is made from a plaster model of the child's entire head. A properly secured helmet effectively utilizes pressure over three areas of suspension and covers the maximum surface area of the cranium and prevent movement:

- anteriorly across the forehead just above the eyebrows
- enclosing the posterior and inferior aspects of the occiput
- around the crest of the mandible and chin.

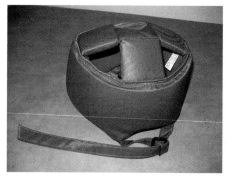

Fig. 13.2 Lightweight soft-fabric helmet for infants.

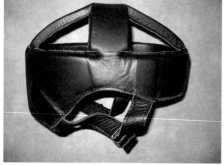

Fig. 13.3 Scrum-type leather-covered padded helmet.

162

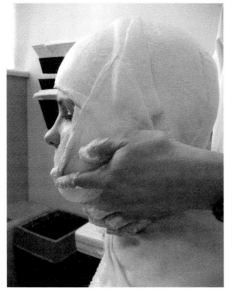

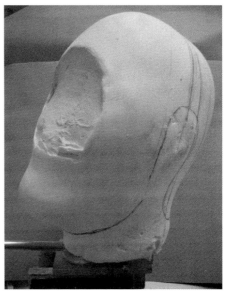

Fig. 13.4 A plaster-cast model of the child's head is the first stage in the fabrication process for a custom-moulded helmet.

Fig. 13.5 Modifications to the positive model are important to ensure proper fit of the helmet.

Moulding the helmet to a model of the child's head ensures a snug and intimate fit, ensures the helmet does not restrict neck flexion or extension, permits full field of vision, and provides more complete protection of the head (Belbin and Giavedoni 1987). Two custom helmet designs with rigid shells currently used at the Bloorview MacMillan Children's Centre Headwear Clinic in Toronto are (1) the custom full-face with the chin incorporated in the helmet, and (2) the cranial cap secured with a chin strap. Both designs have a rigid outer shell and are custom-made from a plaster replica of the cranium. The prescription of a specific helmet is determined during the patient assessment where the diagnosis and individual falling patterns and behaviours are identified through consultation with parents or caregivers (Belbin and Giavedoni 1987).

A negative plaster model of the whole child's head is the first stage in the fabrication process for a custom-moulded helmet (Fig. 13.4). Specific modifications to the positive model are important to ensure proper fit of the helmet (Fig. 13.5):

1) the cast is smoothed over to remove any stockinette lines and major irregularities
2) the area inferior to the occiput is undercut and the posterior aspect of the neck is reduced to contour and provide posterior suspension for the helmet
3) the inferior portion of the chin is flattened and undercut to lock in the chin and reduce bulk to allow for increased neck flexion
4) the anterior trim lines are marked to define the frontal opening of the helmet. Plaster build-ups are added that extend:

- inferiorly from the apex of the forehead
- anteriorly from the apex of the cheek bones on both sides, and
- superiorly from above the crest of the chin.

The full face protective helmet consists of a hinged, hard modified-polyethylene outer shell and incorporates an ethylene vinyl acetate (EVA) foam liner. The liner is vacuum-formed first over the modified plaster positive model of the head in front and back halves (Fig. 13.6). Additional foam is added over the chin and forehead to provide increased protection and clearance for the entire face in the event of a fall forwards on to a flat surface. The outer shell is then drape-formed over the cast and lining (Fig. 13.7). Slots are cut out at the top of the helmet to reduce the weight, provide ventilation, and create a flexible hinge between its anterior and posterior sections for ease of donning and doffing (Fig. 13.8) (Ryan et al.1992).

Helmet trim-lines must ensure the helmet does not restrict neck flexion or extension, therefore the distal posterior trim line must enclose the posterior and inferior aspects of the occiput, and the anterior distal trim-line runs around the crest of the mandible and encloses the chin. The trim-lines around the face must permit the wearer full field of vision, and thus run anteriorly across the forehead just above the eyebrows, and laterally around the eyes to allow full peripheral vision (Fig. 13.9). The plastic is normally cut out around the ears for ventilation and in order not to impair hearing; however, certain clinical conditions may require one or both ears to be covered for additional protection. In such cases, the plastic would not be cut out over the ear, but would be ventilated with holes to reduce heat and maintain some airflow through the helmet. Face masks can be attached to the main shell if required for extra protection (Fig. 13.10).

The cranial cap does not include the chin in the main shell. The cap is constructed in the same way as the full-face design, except that its outer shell consists of a solid piece of polyethylene without a hinge and has ventilation slots at the top, and is secured to the wearer

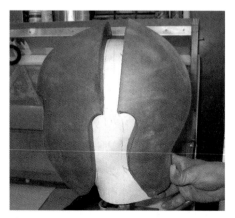

Fig. 13.6 The lining is moulded in EVA as front and back halves.

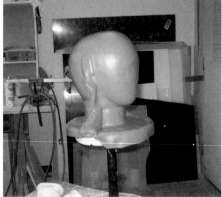

Fig. 13.7 The hard outer shell is moulded in one piece over the cast and lining.

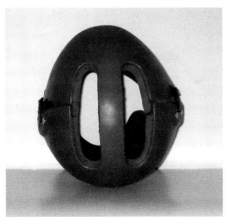

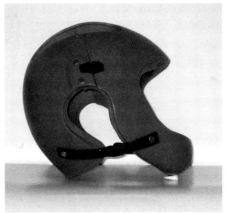

Fig. 13.8 Slots are cut although not at the centre so that a hinge exists between its anterior and posterior sections to ease donning and doffing.

Fig. 13.9 Plastic is trimmed around the face and ears and secured with clips.

with a padded chin strap. Ventilation is the main difficulty, since there is only so much plastic that can be cut away safely to increase air flow to the head and maintain the structural integrity of the helmet.

Helmets may be made to appear more socially and aesthetically acceptable by using patterned or coloured outer shells, custom painting, decals, custom covers, etc. in order to facilitate wearing compliance and minimize social stigmas. One innovation to a rigid custom cranial cap design was the Muckamore Abbey Cosmetic Helmet which incorporated an Irish tweed outer cover with several cap styles. The tweed also provided additional cushioning to the helmet (Barker 1981).

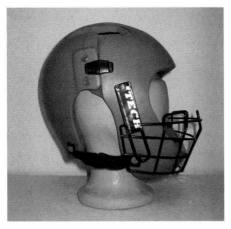

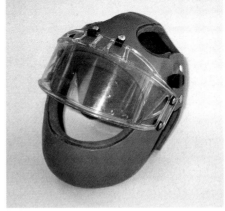

Fig. 13.10 Mouth, eye or full-face protection can be added to the helmet if required.

Corrective headware

The word 'plagiocephaly' comes from the Ancient Greek, and literally means 'oblique or twisted head'. Deformation of the skull can occur in the womb, through the birthing process, following prolonged supine sleeping positioning, or due to tight sternocleidmastoid muscle. There are two main types of plagiocephaly, synostotic and non-synostotic (deformational). In the synostotic case one or more of the sutures are fused and surgery is often necessary as the deformity is likely to increase the risk of raised intracranial pressure. Non-synostotic, deformational or positional plagiocephaly, on the other hand, may respond to conservative management.

The 'Back to Sleep' programme was introduced by the American Academy of Pediatrics in 1992 to discourage parents from placing infants to sleep in prone postures. The incidence of sudden infant death syndrome (SIDS) decreased remarkably by almost 40% following this advice. The programme encourages parents to place infants on their backs when sleeping during the night and at nap times, as well as during the day in infant carriers, car seats and strollers. The period since this advice was introduced has also been associated with an increase in the numbers of infants developing positional plagiocephaly. However, as the deformity is purely aesthetic and to some extent self-resolving, and is not known to impair brain development, decisions about intervention for cosmetic reasons are controversial. Despite the variety in the shapes of adult skulls, today's society is inundated with images that focus on appearance, symmetry and cosmetic beauty for men and women alike. Given such a strong emphasis on facial appearance it is no surprise that many parents seek out aggressive treatment, using a regimen of helmet therapy to remould the skull.

CRANIAL ANATOMY

The infant skull is made of nine bones: two frontal, parietal, occipital and sphenoid bones and one occipital. In between these bones are fibrous structures that allow the various skull bones to distort. This is especially important during the birthing process as well as for rapid brain growth that occurs right after birth. Fontanelles are 'soft spots' that are present at every junction of the parietal bones. The two largest are the anterior and posterior ones that are easily palpable on the young infant. Until these fontanelles and sutures fuse, the skull shape can be deformed by external forces. If they do deform due to a constant external force, such as during the birthing process or sleeping supine, flattened areas or asymmetry may develop. It is important to note that the sutures and fontanelles will fuse at different times through infancy, childhood and adulthood and that these times will vary from one individual to the next.

ASSESSMENT

When it occurs, deformational or positional plagiocephaly will usually be noticed within the first few months of birth. Detection of plagiocephaly is contingent on a number of factors: severity of the impairment, follicular count of the child, and the location of the affected area. For instance, if the cranial deformity is moderate to severe and the infant has very little hair, the parents or physician will readily notice a flattened area and asymmetry. If the deformity is mild, however, and the child has a lot of hair, detecting a flattened area is more difficult. This issue raises the predicament of whether or not to treat children who present mildly with this condition.

TREATMENT OPTIONS

The mechanism of postural deformity in plagiocephaly is analogous to a ball with a flat spot. If the ball is placed on a flat surface it will tend towards the most stable position and rest on the flattened area. Unfortunately, when infants are placed on their backs for long periods of time any flattened area is exacerbated due to the persistent deforming force. Typically, babies under 4 months of age will spend the vast majority of time sleeping or lying down. Infants sleep between 18 and 22 hours a day, and the time they spend awake may be in a car seat, stroller, or cushion for feeding; and without varied position, the consistent force on an infant's skull may easily result in deformation.

From birth to 4 months

Treatment for plagiocephaly is dependent on several factors: age of the child, amount of deformation, parent compliance, and coexisting medical issues. If plagiocephaly is noticed early on, up to approximately 4 months of age, counter-positioning is the recommended mode of treatment. At this youngest age the infant's skull remains very malleable and symmetry of the skull may be achieved without the use of a helmet. Counter-positioning is defined as the use of conservative steps to stop the child from lying on the flattened area. Strategies to accomplish counter-positioning include reducing the time that the infant is lying on the flattened area, using pillows to place the child in more desirable positions, and placing toys and pictures in a position that would encourage the child to turn away from the flattened area. Counter-positioning can be effective at an early age when the infant's musculature is not strong enough to counteract the forces of the various pillows and wedges that are available. However, as the child gets older, the efficacy of these strategies is undermined as they get stronger and are able to switch positions freely while sleeping.

From 4 months to 1 year

Once an infant has gained sufficient motor control to roll and sit independently, it is arguable how ongoing cranial asymmetry should be treated. The child will not now rest on any flattened area for prolonged periods since, with increasing neck control, they will spend increasing amounts of time rolling supine and also sitting more independently. It is not clear whether treatment with counter-positioning should continue or alternative interventions now be considered. There are conflicting studies presented in the literature which makes the information difficult to present to families (Bridges et al. 2002, Persing et al. 2003, Bialocerkowski et al. 2005). Many parents request further intervention using a helmet if they are not satisfied with the results after trying counter-positioning. Using a helmet can be a successful strategy to reshape the orientation of the cranial structure, and it tends to be most effective when started between 5 and 6 months of age. Pressure is maintained on the more prominent areas of the skull while spaces are created in the areas of the flat spot; this removes pressure from the flattened area, thus allowing growth. The transition from counter-positioning strategies to adopting helmet use should be considered when the infant is approximately 5–6 months old. The temporal aspect is paramount as there still is time to influence the shape of the skull before the cranial sutures fuse. Once skull growth is complete and the sutures are fused a helmet can have little or no remoulding effect.

CORRECTIVE HELMET FABRICATION

After plagiocephaly has been recognized as a concern by the parents, family doctor or paediatrician, a consultation may be made with the orthotist. Counter-positioning remains the treatment of choice up to approximately 5 months of age. After helmet treatment has been discussed, parents have to decide if they want to try using a helmet to help re-shape their child's skull. If the parents choose to use a helmet, then measurements and a cast are taken; computer-aided design and manufacture methods also exist. Measurements consist of a circumference around the skull just above the eyebrows and from above eyebrows to the anterior opening of each ear; this is to help determine symmetry of the ears in the frontal plane. Measurements are taken every month for a minimum of 4 months after the child receives the helmet and are used for comparisons with previous assessments.

After taking the measurements, preparations for taking the cast are necessary. Two 4-inch stockinette tubes are cut and stitched in a semicircle and pulled over the child's skull down as far as the neck. A hole is cut out for the eyes, nose and mouth. The ears are marked with an indelible marker and so is the centre of the skull front and back. These markings are important in orienting the positive mould before modifications are made. Next plaster slabs, three layers thick, are wrapped around the skull from just above the eyebrows to the nape of the neck including the ears on either side. Five slabs of plaster are usually required to make the negative plaster-cast. A centre line is drawn on the forehead for orientation when filling the negative with liquid plaster (Fig. 13.11). Two small gaps are left to avoid creating a vacuum and suction effect when removing the cast. Once the negative mould has hardened it is slipped off. It is important not to wait too long before removing the cast

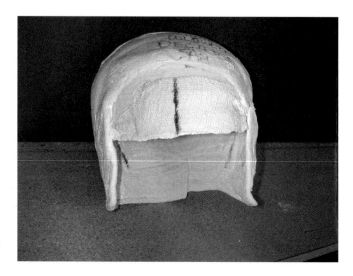

Fig. 13.11 Negative cast of the infant's head.

168

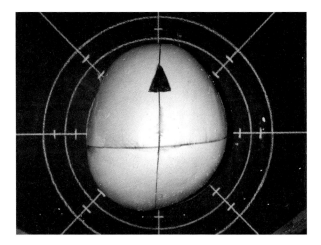

Fig. 13.12 Asymmetry of the head can be assessed by placing the positive cast over concentric circles.

due to heat dissipated as the cast sets, which can raise the infant's internal temperature and lead to various physiological concerns.

Liquid plaster is poured into the negative cast and a mandrel placed in the middle. Once set, this positive cast can be used to assess asymmetry (Fig. 13.12), and can then be modified to create a more symmetrical head shape. Plaster in bossing areas is reduced and build-ups are added to the flat spots and screened to give a smooth finish. The cast is then ready to be moulded. The positive is covered with a nylon stocking. Two foam liners are than heated in the oven and bubble-moulded over the cast. Each liner is composed of ⅜-inch medium durometer EVA which will compress to ¼ inch each after drape moulding. Silicon spray is used between the two bubble-mouldings to prevent the two pieces of foam from adhering to one another. Finally the ¼-inch ABS plastic sheet is heated to 400°C and bubble-moulded over the helmet. In each of the bubble moulds, vacuum is used to ensure an intimate fit between the cast, foam and ABS. After these materials are cooled for approximately 1 hour the helmet is ready to be trimmed for an initial fitting.

The trim-lines of the helmet are kept long, prior to the initial fitting (Fig. 13.13); material is then removed in stages that occur while the child is present until the appropriate trim-lines are achieved. The whole process of trial fitting and trimming to reach the final fit takes approximately 2½ hours. With regard to the anterior aspect, the helmet is at the level of the eyebrows or slightly above. This is important in order to help re-shape the frontal aspect of the skull. In the posterior region the final trim-line will be just below the occipital area. Cupping the occipital is important in order to help stop the helmet from rotating on the infant's skull. Cut-outs are also made for the ears.

Once these trim-lines are achieved a chin strap and posterior tension strap are added as well as holes for ventilation. The tension strap and corresponding slot is made at an angle perpendicular to the flat spot (Fig. 13.14). This is to insure that slight pressure is provided on the high points and none on the flattened area. Parents are shown how to don the helmet on their child and how much tension to use with the posterior strap. It is important that the family try fitting the helmet in the clinic themselves a few times before leaving. A snug but

Fig. 13.13 Corrective helmet ready for trial fitting.

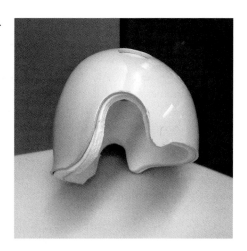

not tight fit is recommended. The chin strap is set to allow for ease of movement of the jaw for eating, and is made of an elastic strapping material to reduce the danger of choking. It anchors the helmet and helps discourage rotation in all planes. Given that the interior of the helmet is symmetrical and the infant's skull is not, slight rotation of the helmet on the skull is inevitable; as the skull re-shapes, however, this becomes less of an issue.

The recommended duration of helmet use is about 4 months, for approximately 20 hours a day. Since plagiocephaly is a largely cosmetic concern, parents or caregivers can decide to terminate the use of the helmet at any time. Disadvantages of the helmet are excessive perspiration and potential pressure problems; there are also social issues for both the child and parents to contend with, as the helmet is immediately visible. The helmet has

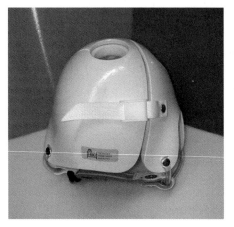
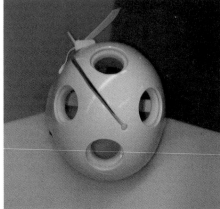

Fig. 13.14 The finished helmet includes a slot and strap to adjust the pressure applied by the helmet, chin strap and ventilation holes.

to be cleaned three times a day with antibacterial soap, and the child's skull also has to be cleaned with water or a mild soap. Problems due to excessive pressure, such as reddening of the skin, may occur on the bulbous areas of the skull; however, these are usually not of concern. If they are, the helmet may be applied to tight or the foam on the interior may have to be eased. Social issues tend to affect parents more than the infants. Fortunately, for the most part, infants appear to adapt quite well to the helmet.

Although the treatment of plagiocephaly using helmets has become increasingly applied in North America, the approach remains less common in the UK, where repositioning and reassurance are predominantly favoured. Several academic reviews highlight the poor evidence to support helmet therapy over repositioning, especially given the high cost of treatment (Bridges et al. 2002, Persing et al. 2003, Bialocerkowski et al. 2005). However one feels sympathy for parents who seek advice regarding the shape of their child's head and then have to make a decision about whether to use helmet therapy when there is only a limited time window in which the intervention can be used.

References

Barker RJ (1981) Construction of the Muckamore Abbey cosmetic helmet for protection of special care patients. *Physiotherapy* **67**: 47–9.
Belbin G, Giavedoni B (1987) Custom-fitted protective headwear. *JACPOC* **22**: 4–7.
Bialocerkowski AE, Vladusic SL, Howell SM (2005) Conservative interventions for positional plagiocephaly: a systematic review. *Dev Med Child Neurol* **47**: 563–70.
Bridges SJ, Chambers TL, Pople IK (2002) Plagiocephaly and head binding. *Arch Dis Child* **86**: 144–5.
Eguchi S, Tokioka T, Motoyoshi A, Wakamura S (1994) A self-controllable mask with helmet to prevent self finger-mutilation in the Lesch–Nyhan syndrome. *Arch Phys Med Rehabil* **75**: 709–10.
McAdam DB, Sherman JA, Sheldon JB, Napolitano DA (2004) Behavioral interventions to reduce the pica of persons with developmental disabilities. *Behavior Modif* **28**: 45–72.
Nyhan WL (1976) Behavior in the Lesch-Nyhan syndrome. *J Autism Child Schiz* **6**: 235–52.
Persing J, James H, Swanson J, Kattwinkel J (2003) Prevention and management of positional skull deformities in infants. American Academy of Pediatrics Committee on Practice and Ambulatory Medicine, Section on Plastic Surgery and Section on Neurological Surgery. *Pediatrics* **112**: 199–202.
Rivara FP, Astley SJ, Clarren SK, Thompson DC, Thompson RS (1999) Fit of bicycle safety helmets and risk of head injuries in children. *Inj Prev* **5**: 194–7.
Ryan S, Belbin G, Slack M, Naumann S, Moran R (1992) Development of a modular design, custom-fitted protective helmet. *JPO* **4**: 213–18.
Sneed RC, Stencel C (2001) Protective helmets for children with special health care needs. *South Med J* **94**: 519–21.

INDEX

179